HUMAN CLONING

AND

HUMAN DIGNITY:

An Ethical Inquiry

THE PRESIDENT'S COUNCIL ON BIOETHICS
WASHINGTON, D.C.
JULY 2002
WWW.BIOETHICS.GOV

Contents

vi

viii

THE PRESIDENT'S COUNCIL ON BIOETHICS
Washington, D.C.

July 10, 2002

The President
The White House
Washington, D.C.

Dear Mr. President:

I am pleased to present to you the first report of the President's Council on Bioethics, *Human Cloning and Human Dignity: An Ethical Inquiry.* The product of six months of discussion, research, reflection, and deliberation, we hope that it will prove a worthy contribution to public understanding of this momentous question.

Man's biotechnological powers are expanding in scope, at what seems an accelerating pace. Many of these powers are double-edged, offering help for human suffering, yet threatening harm to human dignity. Human cloning, we are confident, is but a foretaste—the herald of many dazzling genetic and reproductive technologies that will raise profound moral questions well into the future. It is crucial that we try to understand its full human significance.

We have tried to conduct our inquiry into human cloning unblinkered, with our eyes open not only to the benefits of the new biotechnologies but also to their challenges—moral, social, and political. We have not suppressed differences but sought rather to illuminate them, that all might better appreciate what is at stake. We have eschewed a thin utilitarian calculus of costs and benefits, or a narrow analysis based only on individual "rights." Rather, we have tried to ground our reflections on the broader plane of human procreation and human healing, with their deeper meanings. Seen in this way, we find that the power to clone human beings is not just another in a series of powerful tools for overcoming unwanted infertility or treating disease.

Rather, cloning represents a turning point in human history—the crossing of an important line separating sexual from asexual procreation and the first step toward genetic control over the next generation. It thus carries with it a number of troubling consequences for children, family, and society.

Although the Council is not unanimous, either in some of its ethical conclusions or its policy recommendations, we are unanimous in submitting the entire report as a fair and accurate reflection both of our views and of the state of the question. To summarize our findings briefly:

First. The Council holds unanimously that cloning-to-produce-children is unethical, ought not to be attempted, and should be indefinitely banned by federal law, regardless of who performs the act or whether federal funds are involved.

Second. On the related question of the ethics of cloning-for-biomedical research, the Council is of several minds and is divided in its policy preferences:

- Seven Members (a minority), eager to see the research proceed, recommend permitting cloning-for-biomedical-research to go forward, but only under strict federal regulation.

- Ten Members (a majority), convinced that no human cloning should be permitted at least for the time being, recommend instituting, by law, a four-year ban on cloning-for-biomedical-research, applicable to all researchers regardless of whether federal funds are involved.

Third. The same ten-Member majority recommends a federal review of current and projected practices of human embryo research, pre-implantation genetic diagnosis, genetic modification of human embryos and gametes, and related matters, with a view to recommending and shaping ethically sound policies for the entire field. A thorough federal review, during the moratorium, could help to clarify the issues and foster a public consensus about how to proceed, not just on cloning-for-biomedical-research but on all the related reproductive and genetic technologies. We think this Council is well situated to initiate such a review, and we have already begun it. But we also stand ready to assist any other body that may be established to take up this large and complex subject.

The extensive reasoning underlying these recommendations is given at length in the report and is well summarized in the Executive Summary, and so I shall not rehearse it here.

On behalf of my Council colleagues, and our fine staff, allow me to thank you, Mr. President, for the opportunity you have given us to serve the nation on this weighty subject.

Sincerely,

LEON R. KASS, M.D.
Chairman

Members of the President's Council on Bioethics

LEON R. KASS, M.D., PH.D., *Chairman.*
> Addie Clark Harding Professor, The College and the Committee on Social Thought, University of Chicago. Hertog Fellow, American Enterprise Institute.

ELIZABETH H. BLACKBURN, PH.D., D.SC.
> Professor, Department of Biochemistry and Biophysics, University of California-San Francisco.

STEPHEN L. CARTER, J.D.
> William Nelson Cromwell Professor of Law, Yale Law School.

REBECCA S. DRESSER, J.D., M.S.
> Daniel Noyes Kirby Professor of Law, Washington University School of Law. Professor of Ethics in Medicine, Washington University School of Medicine.

DANIEL W. FOSTER, M.D.
> Donald W. Seldin Distinguished Chair in Internal Medicine, Chairman of the Department of Internal Medicine, University of Texas Southwestern Medical School.

FRANCIS FUKUYAMA, PH.D.
> Bernard Schwartz Professor of International Political Economy, Paul H. Nitze School of Advanced International Studies, Johns Hopkins University.

MICHAEL S. GAZZANIGA, PH.D.
> David T. McLaughlin Distinguished Professor in Cognitive Neuroscience, Director, Center for Cognitive Neuroscience, Dartmouth College.

Council Staff and Consultants

Dean Clancy	Executive Director
Michelle R. Bell	Receptionist/Staff Assistant
Eric Cohen	Senior Research Consultant
Judith Crawford	Administrative Director
Diane M. Gianelli	Director of Communications
Emily Jones	Executive Assistant
Joshua Kleinfeld	Research Analyst
Gabriel Ledeen	Intern
Yuval Levin	Senior Research Analyst
Richard Roblin, Ph.D.	Scientific Director
Megan Suzann Steven	Intern
Brett Swearingen	Intern
Audrea R. Vann	Staff Assistant
Rachel Flick Wildavsky	Director, Education Project
Adam Wolfson	Consultant
Lee L. Zwanziger, Ph.D.	Director of Research

Preface

Human Cloning and Human Dignity: An Ethical Inquiry is the first publication of the President's Council on Bioethics, which was created by President George W. Bush on November 28, 2001, by means of Executive Order 13237.

The Council's purpose is to advise the President on bioethical issues related to advances in biomedical science and technology. In connection with its advisory role, the mission of the Council includes the following functions:

- To undertake fundamental inquiry into the human and moral significance of developments in biomedical and behavioral science and technology.
- To explore specific ethical and policy questions related to these developments.
- To provide a forum for a national discussion of bioethical issues.
- To facilitate a greater understanding of bioethical issues.
- To explore possibilities for useful international collaboration on bioethical issues.

President Bush left the Council free to establish its own priorities among the many issues encompassed within its charter, based on the urgency and gravity of those issues and the public need for practical guidance about them.

The Council had little difficulty in choosing its first topic of inquiry. The ethics of human cloning has been the subject of intense discussion in the United States and throughout the world for more than five years, and it remains the subject of heated debate in Congress. On the surface, discussion has focused on the safety of cloning techniques, the hoped-for medical benefits of cloning research, and the morality of experimenting on human embryos. But driving the conversations are deeper concerns about where biotechnology may be taking us and what it might mean for human freedom, equality, and dignity.

Human cloning, were it to succeed, would enable parents for the first time to determine the entire genetic makeup of their children. Bypassing sexual reproduction, it would move procreation increasingly under artful human control and in the direction of manufacture. Seen as a forerunner of possible future genetic engineering, it raises for many people concerns also about eugenics, the project to "improve" the human race. A world that practiced human cloning, we sense, could be a very different world, perhaps radically different, from the one we know. It is crucial that we try to understand, before it happens, whether, how, and why this may be so.

Investigating human cloning also provides the Council an important opportunity to illustrate how bioethics can and should deal with those technological innovations that touch deeply our humanity. Here, as elsewhere, the most profound issues go beyond the commonplace and utilitarian concerns of feasibility, safety, and efficacy. In addition, on the policy side, cloning offers us a test case for considering whether public control of biotechnology is possible and desirable, and if so, by what means and at what cost.

The Council commenced deliberations on the topic of human cloning at its first meeting in January 2002, and continued the discussion at its February, April, and June meetings, all held in Washington, D.C. We heard presentations on the recent cloning report of the National Academy of Sciences; on human stem cell research, embryonic and adult; on the ethics of embryo research; and on international systems of regulation of embryo research and assisted reproductive technologies. We received a great deal of public comment, oral and written. All told, we held twelve ninety-minute conversations on the subject.

Recognizing "the complex and often competing moral positions" on biomedical issues, President Bush specified in creating the Council that it need not be constrained by "an overriding concern to find consensus." In this report we have chosen not to be so constrained. We have not suppressed disagreements in search of a single, watered-down position. Instead, we have presented clear arguments for the relevant moral and policy positions on multiple sides of these difficult questions, representing each as fairly and fully as we can. As a result, the reader will notice that, on some of the matters discussed in the report, Members of the Council are not all of one mind. Members are united, though, in endorsing the worthiness of the approach taken and the importance of the separate arguments made. Accordingly, the Council is unanimous in owning the entire report and in recommending all its discussions and arguments for serious consideration.

Readers interested in delving further into this subject may wish to consult the Bibliography, which includes all of the documents referred to within the report, and also the verbatim transcripts of our meetings, posted at our website (www.bioethics.gov).

It was in his remarks to the nation on federal funding of embryonic stem cell research, on August 9, 2001, that President Bush first declared his intention to create this Council. At the end of that speech, the President said:

> I will also name a President's council to monitor stem cell research, to recommend appropriate guidelines and regulations, and to consider all of the medical and ethical ramifications of biomedical innovation. . . . This council will keep us apprised of new developments and give our nation a forum to continue to discuss and evaluate these important issues. As we go forward, I hope we will always be guided by both intellect and heart, by both our capabilities and our conscience.

It has been our goal in these pages—and shall remain our goal in the future—to live up to the President's high hopes and noble aspirations.

LEON R. KASS, M.D.
Chairman

Executive Summary

For the past five years, the prospect of human cloning has been the subject of considerable public attention and sharp moral debate, both in the United States and around the world. Since the announcement in February 1997 of the first successful cloning of a mammal (Dolly the sheep), several other species of mammals have been cloned. Although a cloned human child has yet to be born, and although the animal experiments have had low rates of success, the production of functioning mammalian cloned offspring suggests that the eventual cloning of humans must be considered a serious possibility.

In November 2001, American researchers claimed to have produced the first cloned human embryos, though they reportedly reached only a six-cell stage before they stopped dividing and died. In addition, several fertility specialists, both here and abroad, have announced their intention to clone human beings. The United States Congress has twice taken up the matter, in 1998 and again in 2001-2002, with the House of Representatives in July 2001 passing a strict ban on all human cloning, including the production of cloned human embryos. As of this writing, several cloning-related bills are under consideration in the Senate. Many other nations have banned human cloning, and the United Nations is considering an international convention on the subject. Finally, two major national reports have been issued on human reproductive cloning, one by the National Bioethics Advisory Commission (NBAC) in 1997, the other by the National Academy of Sciences (NAS) in January 2002. Both the NBAC and the NAS reports called for further consideration of the ethical and social questions raised by cloning.

The debate over human cloning became further complicated in 1998 when researchers were able, for the first time, to isolate human embryonic stem cells. Many scientists believe that these versatile cells, capable of becoming any type of cell in the body, hold great promise for understanding and treating many chronic diseases and conditions. Some scientists also believe that stem cells derived from *cloned* human embryos, produced explicitly for such research, might prove uniquely useful for studying many genetic diseases and devising novel therapies. Public reaction to the prospect of cloning-for-biomedical-research has been mixed: some Americans support it for its medical promise; others oppose it because it requires the exploitation and destruction of nascent human life, which would be created solely for research purposes.

Human Cloning: What Is at Stake?

The intense attention given to human cloning in both its potential uses, for reproduction as well as for research, strongly suggests that people do not regard it as just another new technology. Instead, we see it as something quite different, something that touches fundamental aspects of our humanity. The notion of cloning raises issues about identity and individuality, the meaning of having children, the difference between procreation and manufacture, and the relationship between the generations. It also raises new questions about the manipulation of some human beings for the benefit of others, the freedom and value of biomedical inquiry, our obligation to heal the sick (and its limits), and the respect and protection owed to nascent human life.

Finally, the legislative debates over human cloning raise large questions about the relationship between science and society, especially about whether society can or should exercise ethical and prudential control over biomedical technology and the conduct of biomedical research. Rarely has such a seemingly small innovation raised such big questions.

The Inquiry: Our Point of Departure

As Members of the President's Council on Bioethics, we have taken up the larger ethical and social inquiry called for in the

NBAC and NAS reports, with the aim of advancing public understanding and informing public policy on the matter. We have attempted to consider human cloning (both for producing children and for biomedical research) within its larger human, technological, and ethical contexts, rather than to view it as an isolated technical development. We focus first on the broad human goods that it may serve as well as threaten, rather than on the immediate impact of the technique itself. By our broad approach, our starting on the plane of human goods, and our open spirit of inquiry, we hope to contribute to a richer and deeper understanding of what human cloning means, how we should think about it, and what we should do about it.

On some matters discussed in this report, Members of the Council are not of one mind. Rather than bury these differences in search of a spurious consensus, we have sought to present all views fully and fairly, while recording our agreements as well as our genuine diversity of perspectives, including our differences on the final recommendations to be made. By this means, we hope to help policymakers and the general public appreciate more thoroughly the difficulty of the issues and the competing goods that are at stake.

Fair and Accurate Terminology

There is today much confusion about the terms used to discuss human cloning, regarding both the activity involved and the entities that result. The Council stresses the importance of striving not only for accuracy but also for fairness, especially because the choice of terms can decisively affect the way questions are posed, and hence how answers are given. We have sought terminology that most accurately conveys the descriptive reality of the matter, in order that the moral arguments can then proceed on the merits. We have resisted the temptation to solve the moral questions by artful redefinition or by denying to some morally crucial element a name that makes clear that there is a moral question to be faced.

On the basis of (1) a careful analysis of the act of cloning, and its relation to the means by which it is accomplished and the purposes it may serve, and (2) an extensive critical examination of alternative terminologies, the Council has adopted the following definitions for the most important terms in the matter of human cloning:

- *Cloning:* A form of reproduction in which offspring result not from the chance union of egg and sperm (sexual reproduction) but from the deliberate replication of the genetic makeup of another single individual (asexual reproduction).

- *Human cloning:* The asexual production of a new human organism that is, at all stages of development, genetically virtually identical to a currently existing or previously existing human being. It would be accomplished by introducing the nuclear material of a human somatic cell (donor) into an oocyte (egg) whose own nucleus has been removed or inactivated, yielding a product that has a human genetic constitution virtually identical to the donor of the somatic cell. (This procedure is known as "somatic cell nuclear transfer," or SCNT). We have declined to use the terms "reproductive cloning" and "therapeutic cloning." We have chosen instead to use the following designations:

- *Cloning-to-produce-children:* Production of a cloned human embryo, formed for the (proximate) purpose of initiating a pregnancy, with the (ultimate) goal of producing a child who will be genetically virtually identical to a currently existing or previously existing individual.

- *Cloning-for-biomedical-research:* Production of a cloned human embryo, formed for the (proximate) purpose of using it in research or for extracting its stem cells, with the (ultimate) goals of gaining scientific knowledge of normal and abnormal development and of developing cures for human diseases.

- *Cloned human embryo:* (a) A human embryo resulting from the nuclear transfer process (as contrasted with a human embryo arising from the union of egg and sperm). (b) The immediate (and developing) product of the initial act of cloning, accomplished by successful SCNT, whether used subsequently in attempts to produce children or in biomedical research.

Scientific Background

Cloning research and stem cell research are being actively investigated and the state of the science is changing rapidly; significant new developments could change some of the interpretations in our report. At present, however, a few general points may be highlighted.

- *The technique of cloning.* The following steps have been used to produce live offspring in the mammalian species that have been successfully cloned. Obtain an egg cell from a female of a mammalian species. Remove its nuclear DNA, to produce an enucleated egg. Insert the nucleus of a donor adult cell into the enucleated egg, to produce a reconstructed egg. Activate the reconstructed egg with chemicals or electric current, to stimulate it to commence cell division. Sustain development of the cloned embryo to a suitable stage in vitro, and then transfer it to the uterus of a female host that has been suitably prepared to receive it. Bring to live birth a cloned animal that is genetically virtually identical (except for the mitochondrial DNA) to the animal that donated the adult cell nucleus.

- *Animal cloning: low success rates, high morbidity.* At least seven species of mammals (none of them primates) have been successfully cloned to produce live births. Yet the production of live cloned offspring is rare and the failure rate is high: more than 90 percent of attempts to initiate a clonal pregnancy do not result in successful live birth. Moreover, the live-born cloned animals suffer high rates of deformity and disability, both at birth and later on. Some biologists attribute these failures to errors or incompleteness of epigenetic reprogramming of the somatic cell nucleus.

- *Attempts at human cloning.* At this writing, it is uncertain whether anyone has attempted cloning-to-produce-children (although at least one physician is now claiming to have initiated several active clonal pregnancies, and others are reportedly working on it). We do not know whether a transferred cloned human embryo can progress all the way to live birth.

- *Stem cell research.* Human embryonic stem cells have been isolated from embryos (produced by IVF) at the blastocyst stage or from the germinal tissue of fetuses. Human adult stem (or multipotent) cells have been isolated from a variety of tissues. Such cell populations can be differentiated in vitro into a number of different cell types, and are currently being studied intensely for their possible uses in regenerative medicine. Most scientists working in the field believe that stem cells (both embryonic and adult) hold great promise as routes toward cures and treatments for many human diseases and disabilities. All stem cell research is at a very early stage, and it is too soon to tell which approaches will prove most useful, and for which diseases.

- *The transplant rejection problem.* To be effective as long-term treatments, cell transplantation therapies will have to overcome the immune rejection problem. Cells and tissues derived from *adult* stem cells and returned to the patient from whom they were taken would not be subject (at least in principle) to immune rejection.

- *Stem cells from cloned embryos.* Human embryonic stem cell preparations could potentially be produced by using somatic cell nuclear transfer to produce a cloned human embryo, and then taking it apart at the blastocyst stage and isolating stem cells. These stem cells would be genetically virtually identical to cells from the nucleus donor, and thus could potentially be of great value in biomedical research. Very little work of this sort has been done to date in animals, and there are as yet no *published* reports of cloned *human* embryos grown to the blastocyst stage. Although the promise of such research is at this time unknown, most researchers believe it will yield very useful and important knowledge, pointing toward new therapies and offering one of several possible routes to circumvent the immune rejection problem. Although some experimental results in animals are indeed encouraging, they also demonstrate some tendency even of cloned stem cells to stimulate an immune response.

- *The fate of embryos used in research.* All extractions of stem cells from human embryos, cloned or not, involve the destruction of these embryos.

The Ethics of Cloning-to-Produce-Children

Two separate national-level reports on human cloning (NBAC, 1997; NAS, 2002) concluded that attempts to clone a human being would be unethical at this time due to safety concerns and the likelihood of harm to those involved. The Council concurs in this conclusion. But we have extended the work of these distinguished bodies by undertaking a broad ethical examination of the merits of, and difficulties with, cloning-to-produce-children.

Cloning-to-produce-children might serve several purposes. It might allow infertile couples or others to have genetically-related children; permit couples at risk of conceiving a child with a genetic disease to avoid having an afflicted child; allow the bearing of a child who could become an ideal transplant donor for a particular patient in need; enable a parent to keep a living connection with a dead or dying child or spouse; or enable individuals or society to try to "replicate" individuals of great talent or beauty. These purposes have been defended by appeals to the goods of freedom, existence (as opposed to nonexistence), and well-being—all vitally important ideals.

A major weakness in these arguments supporting cloning-to-produce-children is that they overemphasize the freedom, desires, and control of parents, and pay insufficient attention to the well-being of the cloned child-to-be. The Council holds that, once the child-to-be is carefully considered, these arguments are not sufficient to overcome the powerful case against engaging in cloning-to-produce-children.

First, cloning-to-produce-children would violate the principles of the ethics of human research. Given the high rates of morbidity and mortality in the cloning of other mammals, we believe that cloning-to-produce-children would be extremely unsafe, and that attempts to produce a cloned child would be highly unethical. Indeed, our moral analysis of this matter leads us to conclude that this is not, as is sometimes implied, a merely temporary objection, easily removed by the improvement of technique. We offer reasons for believing that the safety risks might be enduring, and offer arguments in support of a strong conclusion: that conducting experiments in an effort to make cloning-to-produce-children less dangerous would itself be an unacceptable violation of the norms of research ethics. *There seems to be no ethical way to try to discover whether cloning-to-produce-children can become safe, now or in the future.*

If carefully considered, the concerns about safety also begin to reveal the ethical principles that should guide a broader assessment of cloning-to-produce-children: the principles of freedom, equality, and human dignity. To appreciate the broader human significance of cloning-to-produce-children, one needs first to reflect on the meaning of having children; the meaning of asexual, as opposed to sexual, reproduction; the importance of origins and genetic endowment for identity and sense of self; the meaning of exercising greater human control over the processes and "products" of human reproduction; and the difference between begetting and making. Reflecting on these topics, the Council has identified five categories of concern regarding cloning-to-produce-children. (Different Council Members give varying moral weight to these different concerns.)

- *Problems of identity and individuality.* Cloned children may experience serious problems of identity both because each will be genetically virtually identical to a human being who has already lived and because the expectations for their lives may be shadowed by constant comparisons to the life of the "original."
- *Concerns regarding manufacture.* Cloned children would be the first human beings whose entire genetic makeup is

selected in advance. They might come to be considered more like products of a designed manufacturing process than "gifts" whom their parents are prepared to accept as they are. Such an attitude toward children could also contribute to increased commercialization and industrialization of human procreation.

- *The prospect of a new eugenics.* Cloning, if successful, might serve the ends of privately pursued eugenic enhancement, either by avoiding the genetic defects that may arise when human reproduction is left to chance, or by preserving and perpetuating outstanding genetic traits, including the possibility, someday in the future, of using cloning to perpetuate genetically engineered enhancements.

- *Troubled family relations.* By confounding and transgressing the natural boundaries between generations, cloning could strain the social ties between them. Fathers could become "twin brothers" to their "sons"; mothers could give birth to their genetic twins; and grandparents would also be the "genetic parents" of their grandchildren. Genetic relation to only one parent might produce special difficulties for family life.

- *Effects on society.* Cloning-to-produce-children would affect not only the direct participants but also the entire society that allows or supports this activity. Even if practiced on a small scale, it could affect the way society looks at children and set a precedent for future nontherapeutic interventions into the human genetic endowment or novel forms of control by one generation over the next. In the absence of wisdom regarding these matters, prudence dictates caution and restraint.

Conclusion: For some or all of these reasons, the Council is in full agreement that cloning-to-produce-children is not only unsafe but also morally unacceptable, and ought not to be attempted.

The Ethics of Cloning-for-Biomedical-Research

Ethical assessment of cloning-for-biomedical-research is far more vexing. On the one hand, such research could lead to important knowledge about human embryological development and gene action, both normal and abnormal, ultimately resulting in treatments and cures for many dreaded illnesses and disabilities. On the other hand, the research is morally controversial because it involves the deliberate production, use, and ultimate destruction of cloned human embryos, and because the cloned embryos produced for research are no different from those that could be implanted in attempts to produce cloned children. The difficulty is compounded by what are, for now, unanswerable questions as to whether the research will in fact yield the benefits hoped for, and whether other promising and morally nonproblematic approaches might yield comparable benefits. The Council, reflecting the differences of opinion in American society, is divided regarding the ethics of research involving (cloned) embryos. *Yet we agree that all parties to the debate have concerns vital to defend, vital not only to themselves but to all of us. No human being and no society can afford to be callous to the needs of suffering humanity, or cavalier about the treatment of nascent human life, or indifferent to the social effects of adopting one course of action rather than another.*

To make clear to all what is at stake in the decision, Council Members have presented, as strongly as possible, the competing ethical cases for and against cloning-for-biomedical-research in the form of first-person attempts at moral suasion. Each case has tried to address what is owed to suffering humanity, to the human embryo, and to the broader society. Within each case, supporters of the position in question speak only for themselves, and not for the Council as a whole.

A. The Moral Case for Cloning-for-Biomedical-Research

The moral case for cloning-for-biomedical-research rests on our obligation to try to relieve human suffering, an obligation that falls most powerfully on medical practitioners and biomedical researchers. We who support cloning-for-biomedical-research all agree that it may offer uniquely useful ways of investigating and possibly treating many chronic debilitating diseases and disabilities, providing aid and relief to millions. We also believe that the moral objections to this research are outweighed by the great good that may come from it. Up to this point, we who support this research all agree. But we differ among ourselves regarding the weight of the moral objections, owing to differences about the moral status of the cloned embryo. These differences of opinion are sufficient to warrant distinguishing two different moral positions within the moral case for cloning-for-biomedical-research:

Position Number One. Most Council Members who favor cloning-for-biomedical-research do so with serious moral concerns. Speaking only for ourselves, we acknowledge the following difficulties, but think that they can be addressed by setting proper boundaries.

- *Intermediate moral status.* While we take seriously concerns about the treatment of nascent human life, we believe there are sound moral reasons for not regarding the embryo in its earliest stages as the moral equivalent of a human person. We believe the embryo has a developing and intermediate moral worth that commands our special respect, but that it is morally permissible to use early-stage cloned human embryos in important research under strict regulation.

- *Deliberate creation for use.* We believe that concerns over the problem of deliberate creation of cloned embryos for use in research have merit, but when properly understood should not preclude cloning-for-biomedical-research. These embryos would not be "created for destruction," but for use in the service of life and medicine. They would be destroyed in the service of a great good, and this should not be obscured.

- *Going too far.* We acknowledge the concern that some researchers might seek to develop cloned embryos beyond the blastocyst stage, and for those of us who believe that the cloned embryo has a developing and intermediate moral status, this is a very real worry. We approve, there-fore, only of research on cloned embryos that is strictly limited to the first fourteen days of development—a point near when the primitive streak is formed and be-fore organ differentiation occurs.

- *Other moral hazards.* We believe that concerns about the exploitation of women and about the risk that cloning-for-biomedical-research could lead to cloning-to-produce-children can be adequately addressed by appro-priate rules and regulations. These concerns need not frighten us into abandoning an important avenue of re-search.

Position Number Two. A few Council Members who favor cloning-for-biomedical-research do not share all the ethical qualms ex-pressed above. Speaking only for ourselves, we hold that this re-search, at least for the purposes presently contemplated, presents no special moral problems, and therefore should be endorsed with enthusiasm as a potential new means of gaining knowledge to serve humankind. Because we accord no special moral status to the early-stage cloned embryo and believe it should be treated essentially like all other human cells, we believe that the moral is-sues involved in this research are no different from those that accompany any biomedical research. What is required is the usual commitment to high standards for the quality of research, scientific integrity, and the need to obtain informed consent from donors of the eggs and somatic cells used in nuclear trans-fer.

B.   The Moral Case against Cloning-for-Biomedical-Research

The moral case against cloning-for-biomedical-research ac-knowledges the possibility—though purely speculative at the moment—that medical benefits might come from this particular avenue of experimentation. But we believe it is morally wrong to exploit and destroy developing human life, even for good rea-sons, and that it is unwise to open the door to the many undesir-able consequences that are likely to result from this research. We find it disquieting, even somewhat ignoble, to treat what are in fact seeds of the next generation as mere raw material for satisfying the needs of our own. Only for very serious reasons should progress toward increased knowledge and medical advances be slowed. But we believe that in this case such reasons are apparent.

- *Moral status of the cloned embryo.* We hold that the case for treating the early-stage embryo as simply the moral equivalent of all other human cells (Position Number Two, above) is simply mistaken: it denies the continuous history of human individuals from the embryonic to fetal to infant stages of existence; it misunderstands the meaning of potentiality; and it ignores the hazardous moral precedent that the routinized creation, use, and destruction of nascent human life would establish. We hold that the case for according the human embryo "intermediate and developing moral status" (Position Number One, above) is also unconvincing, for reasons both biological and moral. Attempts to ground the limited measure of respect owed to a maturing embryo in certain of its developmental features do not succeed, and the invoking of a "special respect" owed to nascent human life seems to have little or no operative meaning if cloned embryos may be created in bulk and used routinely with impunity. If from one perspective the view that the embryo seems to amount to little may invite a weakening of our respect, from another perspective its seeming insignificance should awaken in us a sense of shared humanity and a special obligation to protect it.

- *The exploitation of developing human life.* To engage in cloning-for-biomedical-research requires the irreversible crossing of a very significant moral boundary: the creation of human life expressly and exclusively for the purpose of its use in research, research that necessarily involves its deliberate destruction. If we permit this research to proceed, we will effectively be endorsing the complete transformation of nascent human life into nothing more than a resource or a tool. Doing so would coarsen our moral sensibilities and make us a different society: one less humble toward that which we cannot fully understand, less willing to extend the boundaries of human respect ever outward, and more willing to transgress moral boundaries once it appears to be in our own interests to do so.

- *Moral harm to society.* Even those who are uncertain about the precise moral status of the human embryo have sound ethical-prudential reasons to oppose cloning-for-biomedical-research. Giving moral approval to such research risks significant moral harm to our society by (1) crossing the boundary from sexual to asexual reproduction, thus approving in principle the genetic manipulation and control of nascent human life; (2) opening the door to other moral hazards, such as cloning-to-produce-children or research on later-stage human embryos and fetuses; and (3) potentially putting the federal government in the novel and unsavory position of mandating the destruction of nascent human life. Because we are concerned not only with the fate of the cloned embryos but also with where this research will lead our society, we think prudence requires us not to engage in this research.

- *What we owe the suffering.* We are certainly not deaf to the voices of suffering patients; after all, each of us already shares or will share in the hardships of mortal life. We and our loved ones are all patients or potential patients. But we are not only patients, and easing suffering is not our only moral obligation. As much as we wish to alleviate suffering now and to leave our children a world where suffering can be more effectively relieved, we also want to leave them a world in which we and they want to live—a world that honors moral limits, that respects all life whether strong or weak, and that refuses to secure the good of some human beings by sacrificing the lives of others.

Public Policy Options

The Council recognizes the challenges and risks of moving from moral assessment to public policy. Reflections on the "social contract" between science and society highlight both the importance of scientific freedom and the need for boundaries. We note that other countries often treat human cloning in the context of a broad area of biomedical technology, at the intersection of reproductive technology, embryo research, and genetics, while the public policy debate in the United States has treated cloning largely on its own. We recognize the special difficulty in formulating sound public policy in this area, given that the two ethically distinct matters—cloning-to-produce-children and cloning-for-biomedical-research—will be mutually affected or implicated in any attempts to legislate about either. Nevertheless, our ethical and policy analysis leads us to the conclusion that some deliberate public policy at the federal level is needed in the area of human cloning.

We reviewed the following seven possible policy options and considered their relative strengths and weaknesses: (1) Professional self-regulation but no federal legislative action ("self-regulation"); (2) A ban on cloning-to-produce-children, with neither endorsement nor restriction of cloning-for-biomedical-research ("ban plus silence"); (3) A ban on cloning-to-produce-children, with regulation of the use of cloned embryos for biomedical research ("ban plus regulation"); (4) Governmental regulation, with no legislative prohibitions ("regulation of both"); (5) A ban on all human cloning, whether to produce children or for biomedical research ("ban on both"); (6) A ban on cloning-to-produce-children, with a moratorium or temporary ban on cloning-for-biomedical-research ("ban plus moratorium"); or (7) A moratorium or temporary ban on all human cloning, whether to produce children or for biomedical research ("moratorium on both").

The Council's Policy Recommendations

Having considered the benefits and drawbacks of each of these options, and taken into account our discussions and reflections throughout this report, the Council recommends two possible policy alternatives, each supported by a portion of the Members.

Majority Recommendation: Ten Members of the Council recommend *a ban on cloning-to-produce-children combined with a four-year moratorium on cloning-for-biomedical-research. We also call for a federal review of current and projected practices of human embryo research, pre-implantation genetic diagnosis, genetic modification of human embryos and gametes, and related matters, with a view to recommending and shaping ethically sound policies for the entire field.* Speaking only for ourselves, those of us who support this recommendation do so for some or all of the following reasons:

- By permanently banning cloning-to-produce-children, this policy gives force to the strong ethical verdict against cloning-to-produce-children, unanimous in this Council (and in Congress) and widely supported by the American people. And by enacting a four-year moratorium on the creation of cloned embryos, it establishes an additional safeguard not afforded by policies that would allow the production of cloned embryos to proceed without delay.

- It calls for and provides time for further democratic deliberation about cloning-for-biomedical research, a subject about which the nation is divided and where there remains great uncertainty. A national discourse on this subject has not yet taken place in full, and a moratorium, by making it impossible for either side to cling to the status-quo, would force both to make their full case before the public. By banning all cloning for a time, it allows us to seek moral consensus on whether or not we should cross a major moral boundary (creating nascent cloned human life solely for research) and prevents our crossing it without deliberate decision. It would afford time for scientific evidence, now sorely lacking, to be gathered—from animal models and other avenues of human research—that might give us a better sense of whether cloning-for-biomedical-research would work as promised, and whether other morally non-problematic approaches might be available. It would promote a fuller and better-informed public debate. And it would show respect for the deep moral concerns of the large number of Americans who have serious ethical objections to this research.

- Some of us hold that cloning-for-biomedical-research can never be ethically pursued, and endorse a moratorium to enable us to continue to make our case in a democratic way. Others of us support the moratorium because it would provide the time and incentive required to develop a system of national regulation that might come into use if, at the end of the four-year period, the moratorium were not reinstated or made permanent. Such a system could not be developed overnight, and therefore even those who support the research but want it regulated should see that at the very least a pause is required. In the absence of a moratorium, few proponents of the research would have much incentive to institute an effective regulatory system. Moreover, the very process of proposing such regulations would clarify the moral and prudential judgments involved in deciding whether and how to proceed with this research.

- A moratorium on cloning-for-biomedical-research would enable us to consider this activity in the larger context of research and technology in the areas of developmental biology, embryo research, and genetics, and to pursue a more comprehensive federal regulatory system for setting and executing policy in the entire area.

- Finally, we believe that a moratorium, rather than a lasting ban, signals a high regard for the value of biomedical research and an enduring concern for patients and families whose suffering such research may help alleviate. It would reaffirm the principle that science can progress while upholding the community's moral norms, and would therefore reaffirm the community's moral support for science and biomedical technology.

The decision before us is of great importance. Creating cloned embryos for *any* purpose requires crossing a major moral boundary, with grave risks and likely harms, and once we cross it there will be no turning back. Our society should take the time to make a judgment that is well-informed and morally sound, respectful of strongly held views, and representative of the priorities and principles of the American people. We believe this ban-plus-moratorium proposal offers the best means of achieving these goals.

This position is supported by Council Members Rebecca S. Dresser, Francis Fukuyama, Robert P. George, Mary Ann

Glendon, Alfonso Gómez-Lobo, William B. Hurlbut, Leon R. Kass, Charles Krauthammer, Paul McHugh, and Gilbert C. Meilaender.

Minority Recommendation: Seven Members of the Council recommend *a ban on cloning-to-produce-children, with regulation of the use of cloned embryos for biomedical research.* Speaking only for ourselves, those of us who support this recommendation do so for some or all of the following reasons:

- By permanently banning cloning-to-produce-children, this policy gives force to the strong ethical verdict against cloning-to-produce-children, unanimous in this Council (and in Congress) and widely supported by the American people. We believe that a ban on the transfer of cloned embryos to a woman's uterus would be a sufficient and effective legal safeguard against the practice.

- *It approves cloning-for-biomedical-research and permits it to proceed without substantial delay.* This is the most important advantage of this proposal. The research shows great promise, and its actual value can only be determined by allowing it to go forward now. Regardless of how much time we allow it, no amount of experimentation with animal models can provide the needed understanding of *human* diseases. The special benefits from working with stem cells from *cloned* human embryos cannot be obtained using embryos obtained by IVF. We believe this research could provide relief to millions of Americans, and that the government should therefore support it, within sensible limits imposed by regulation.

- It would establish, *as a condition of proceeding*, the necessary regulatory protections to avoid abuses and misuses of cloned embryos. These regulations might touch on the secure handling of embryos, licensing and prior review of research projects, the protection of egg donors, and the provision of equal access to benefits.

- Some of us also believe that mechanisms to regulate cloning-for-biomedical-research should be part of a larger regulatory program governing all research involving human embryos, and that the federal government should initiate a review of present and projected practices of human embryo research, with the aim of establishing reasonable policies on the matter.

Permitting cloning-for-biomedical-research now, while governing it through a prudent and sensible regulatory regime, is the most appropriate way to allow important research to proceed while insuring that abuses are prevented. We believe that the legitimate concerns about human cloning expressed throughout this report are sufficiently addressed by this ban-plus-regulation proposal, and that the nation should affirm and support the responsible effort to find treatments and cures that might help many who are suffering.

This position is supported by Council Members Elizabeth H. Blackburn, Daniel W. Foster, Michael S. Gazzaniga, William F. May, Janet D. Rowley, Michael J. Sandel, and James Q. Wilson.

Chapter One

The Meaning of Human Cloning: An Overview

The prospect of human cloning[*] burst into the public consciousness in 1997, following the announcement of the successful cloning of Dolly the sheep. It has since captured much attention and generated great debate, both in the United States and around the world. Many are repelled by the idea of producing children who would be genetically virtually identical to pre-existing individuals, and believe such a practice unethical. But some see in such cloning the possibility to do good for infertile couples and the broader society. Some want to outlaw it, and many nations have done so. Others believe the benefits outweigh the risks and the moral concerns, or they oppose legislative interference with science and technology in the name of freedom and progress.

Complicating the national dialogue about human cloning is the isolation in 1998 of human embryonic stem cells, which many scientists believe to hold great promise for understanding and treating many chronic diseases and conditions. Some scientists also believe that stem cells derived from cloned human embryos, produced explicitly for such research, might prove to be uniquely useful for studying many genetic diseases and devising novel therapies. Public reaction to this prospect has been mixed,

---

[*] The term "human cloning" is used in this chapter to refer to all human cloning: cloning-to-produce-children and cloning-for-biomedical-research. When only one particular use of human cloning is intended, we use the more specific term. A full discussion of our choice of terminology is provided in Chapter Three.

with some Americans supporting it in the hope of advancing biomedical research and helping the sick and the suffering, while others are concerned about the instrumentalization or abuse of nascent human life and the resulting danger of moral insensitivity and degradation.

In the United States, several attempts have been made to initiate a comprehensive public review of the significance of human cloning and to formulate appropriate policies. Most notably, the National Bioethics Advisory Commission (NBAC) released a report on the subject of cloning-to-produce-children in 1997.* The Commission concluded that cloning-to-produce-children was, at least for the time being, unethical on safety grounds, and that the deeper and more permanent moral concerns surrounding the practice should be the subject of continuing deliberation "in order to further our understanding of the ethical and social implications of this technology and to enable society to produce appropriate long-term policies regarding this technology" (p. 106).

In this report, the President's Council on Bioethics takes up this important charge, and considers the ethical and social implications of human cloning (both for producing children and for biomedical research) in their full scope, with the aim of informing public policy on the matter.

Our work toward this end is guided by a number of explicit methodological choices about modes of approach, points of departure, and spirit of inquiry. We locate human cloning within its larger human and technological context, rather than consider it in isolation. We focus first on the broad human goods that it may serve or threaten, rather than on the immediate impact of the technique itself. And we present the strongest arguments for the relevant moral and policy positions, rather than frame the arguments in order to seek consensus. By our broad approach, our

---

* *Cloning Human Beings*, Rockville, MD: National Bioethics Advisory Commission, 1997. Human embryonic stem cells had not yet been isolated at the time of the NBAC report, so the Commission did not offer any recommendations on cloning-for-biomedical-research.

starting on the plane of human goods, and our open spirit of inquiry, we hope to contribute to a richer and deeper understanding of what human cloning entails, how we should think about it, and what we should do about it.

Two points of clarification before we proceed. First, all of our considerations and arguments assume that cloning techniques, both for producing children and for providing embryos useful in biomedical research, could succeed in human beings as they have with other mammals. Cloning-to-produce-children has never been successfully carried out in humans, and cloning embryos for biomedical research has not progressed beyond the earliest experiments. We consider it part of our task to judge whether even attempts at human cloning would be ethical or should be lawful. To conduct the analysis and assessment needed for such judgment, we necessarily proceed on the assumption, which we believe is supported by evidence from animal experiments, that human cloning is indeed a possibility—that sooner or later, if it were allowed and attempted, human cloning could be successfully carried out. Practically all public discussion of the ethics of human cloning has, whether expressly or not, proceeded on this same premise, and rightly so.

Second, on some of the matters discussed in this report, Members of the Council are not of one mind. Given that competing goods are at stake, and different people regard them differently, this is not at all surprising. Rather than bury these differences in search of a spurious consensus, we have sought to present all views fairly and fully. Yet transcending these differences is a more fundamental agreement about the worthiness of the approach we have adopted and the arguments we have made. Accordingly, the Council is unanimous in owning the entire report and in recommending, to all, the report's discussions and arguments for serious consideration.

In the remainder of this overview, we describe the context of human cloning and the discussions it has generated. In the course of doing so, we identify the kinds of questions and concerns that would permit a full assessment of the meaning of human cloning. These questions and concerns will guide us throughout the report.

Human Cloning in Context

It is useful to begin by observing how it is that the question of human cloning has come before us. The prospect of cloning human beings confronts us now not as the result of a strong public demand or a long-standing need. Unlike sought-for medical therapies, it was not at the outset pursued as a cure for disease. Neither has it been sought explicitly as a tool for genetic control or "enhancement" of human offspring. Cloning has arisen not so much because it was actively sought for its own sake, but because it is a natural extension of certain biotechnological advances of the past several decades.[*]

For more than half a century, and at an accelerating pace, biomedical scientists have been gaining wondrous new knowledge of the workings of living beings, from small to great. Increasingly, they also are providing precise and sophisticated knowledge of the workings of the human body and mind. Such knowledge of how things work often leads to new technological powers to control or alter these workings, powers ordinarily sought in order to treat human disease and relieve suffering.

Questions regarding the meaning of acquiring such powers—both the promise and the peril—have attracted scholarly and public attention. For more than thirty years, ethical issues related to biomedical advance have occupied the growing field of bioethics. Increasingly, these ethical issues have spawned public discussion and debates. A growing number of people sense that something new and momentous is happening; that the accelerating waves of biotechnical advances touch deeply on our most human concerns; and that the centuries-old project for human

---

[*] Chapter Two summarizes selected historical aspects of the emergence of cloning research and public reactions to the prospect of human cloning. Chapter Four summarizes selected aspects of the current state of the relevant science and technology.

mastery of nature may now be, so to speak, coming home, giving humanity the power to alter and "master" itself.

One important aspect of human life already affected by new biotechnologies is human reproduction. For several decades now, building on advances in genetics, cell biology, and developmental biology, and on technologies used first in animal husbandry, scientists around the world have been adapting techniques and developing tools to study, influence, and manipulate the origins of human life. Beginning with techniques of artificial insemination and progressing through in vitro fertilization (IVF) and intracytoplasmic sperm injection, artificial aids to reproduction have come into standard medical use.

Cloning is, in one sense, another step along this path. It developed as the result of research into mammalian reproduction and development, where it is desired also as a means of replicating animals especially useful to human beings. It is also proposed as an additional means to overcome infertility in humans.

But the controversy surrounding human cloning, and the widespread sense of disquiet and concern with which the prospect has been received around the world, make it clear that cloning is not just another reproductive technology, to be easily assimilated into ordinary life. Nearly all participants in the public debate over human cloning appear to agree that the subject touches upon some of the most fundamental questions regarding the nature of our humanity and the character of our society. In addition, it raises questions about the aims of biomedical science and about the relation between science and society, including the possibility and desirability of exercising public control over the uses of biomedical technology and the conduct of biomedical research. It is because we sense these larger entailments that the subject of cloning matters so much to us. It is these considerations that give the present debate its force and prominence. Thus only through a serious reflection on these broader questions can the full meaning of human cloning be discovered. The prospect of human cloning may have been brought before us by the march of biotechnology, but now that it is here it is incumbent upon us to look well beyond its technical and medical aspects, if we are to appreciate its significance in full.

Three areas of inquiry in particular seem essential to any understanding of the full meaning of human cloning: the nature and meaning of human procreation; the aims, ends, and means of biomedical science and technology; and the relation of science and technology to the larger society.

Cloning and Human Procreation

Human procreation provides the major context for considering the prospect of cloning, especially cloning-to-produce-children. Much of the time, most of us tend to take for granted this central aspect of human life, through which all of us come to be and through which we give birth to our posterity. But the prospect of creating children by cloning brings this subject sharply before us and compels us to examine the nature and meaning of human procreation. For cloning-to-produce-children, while it may be a potential aid to human reproduction, appears also to be a substitute for it, or at least for its natural, un-programmed, sexual character. Properly to assess the meaning of producing cloned children, one must first of all consider the meaning of human procreation in all its aspects and entailments.*

Human procreation, though seemingly an exclusively private act, has a profoundly public meaning. It determines the relations between one generation and the next, shapes identities, creates attachments, and sets up responsibilities for the care and rearing of children (and the care of aging parents or other needy kin). Thus, in considering proposals to clone children, we must ask ourselves what cloning would mean not only for the individual

---

* In order to be sure that we explore fully the human meaning of cloning, we shall examine it in comparison with natural unaided human reproduction, rather than assisted reproduction, say, with in vitro fertilization. The established reproductive technologies do provide some useful points of comparison, but they cannot be taken as the most helpful baseline for understanding the significance of cloning. For that, normal sexual reproduction is the appropriate basis of comparison.

parents and children involved, but also for the surrounding families and for all of society. Opinions on this subject will of course differ, sometimes widely, as they rest on possibly differing perceptions of human procreation and family life. Yet the following basic observations, concerns, and questions seem pertinent, notwithstanding possible differences of opinion among us about how much weight to give them.

Among the important aspects of the topic are these: the meaning of having children; the meaning of sexual, as opposed to asexual, reproduction; the meaning of origins and genetic endowment for identity and sense of self; the meaning of exercising greater human control over the processes and "products" of human reproduction; and the difference between begetting and making.

To understand what it would mean to clone a child, we do well to consider most generally what it means to bring a child into the world, and with what attitude we should regard his or her arrival and presence. Our children are, to begin with, our replacements, those who will one day stand in our place. They are, as Hans Jonas has remarked, "life's own answer to mortality." Though their conception is the fruit of our activity, and though we are responsible for saying "yes" to their arrival, we do not, in normal procreation, command their conception, control their makeup, or rule over their development and birth. They are, in an important sense, "given" to us. Though they are *our* children, they are not our *property*. Though they are our flesh and blood, and deeply kin, they are also independent "strangers" who arrive suddenly out of the darkness and whom we must struggle to get to know. Though we may seek to have them for our own self-fulfillment, they exist also and especially for their own sakes. Though we seek to educate them, they are not like our other projects, determined strictly according to our plans and serving only our desires.

If these observations are correct, certain things follow regarding the attitudes we should have toward our children. We treat them rightly when we treat them as gifts rather than as products, and when we treat them as independent beings whom we are duty-bound to protect and nurture rather than as extensions of ourselves subject only to our wills and whims. Might these attitudes toward children be altered by cloning, and, if so, how? Would social attitudes toward children change, even if cloning were not practiced widely? What might these changes mean?

To understand how the introduction of *a*sexual reproduction might affect human life, we must first seek the intrinsic meaning of the *sexual* character of human reproduction and what it implies for individuals, for families, and for the relation between the generations. Once again, the following observations—while hardly exhaustive—seem pertinent and important.

In sexual reproduction,* each child has two complementary biological progenitors. Each child thus stems from and unites exactly two lineages, lines that trace backward in similar branching fashion for ages. Moreover, the precise genetic endowment of each child is determined by a combination of nature and chance, not by human design: each human child naturally acquires and shares the common human species genotype, each child is genetically (equally) kin to each (both) parent(s), yet each child is also genetically unique.† Cloning-to-produce-children departs from this pattern. A cloned child has unilineal, not bilineal, descent; he or she is genetically kin to only one progenitor. What is more, the genetic kinship is near-total: the cloned child is not genetically unique, but shares almost completely the genetic endowment of the "original" progenitor. Finally, this endowment

---

* The term "sexual reproduction" has two related meanings: the first refers to the act of sexual intercourse that initiates conception by introducing sperm into a woman's generative tract; the second refers to the conception itself, the combination of genetic material from egg and sperm that results in a new organism with a unique genotype. Assisted reproduction techniques like IVF do not involve the former, but do involve the latter and are therefore still rightly considered sexual reproduction. (Likewise, children who are adopted are the fruit of sexual reproduction.) Cloning involves neither, and is therefore described as "asexual reproduction." The second and more fundamental meaning of "*sexual* reproduction," the union of egg and sperm that results in a new genetically unique organism, is the basis of our discussion in this section.

† The apparent exception of identical twins is discussed in Chapter Five.

comes to the cloned child not by chance but by human choice and decision. What do these differences mean for the cloned child, for family relations, and for relations across the generations?

Origins and genetic endowment are significant aspects of who one is and how one regards oneself, of one's "identity," individuality, and place in the social order. The biological linkages and prospects implicit in sexual reproduction help to define us, though, it should go without saying, they do not define us completely. While we are more "what we choose to become" than we are "where we came from," our human beginnings matter, biologically, psychically, and socially. Because of the way we are generated, each of us is at once (1) equally human, (2) equally marked by and from birth as mortal, (3) equally enmeshed in a particular familial nexus of origin, (4) equally individuated in our trajectory from the beginning to the end of our lives—and, if all goes well, (5) equally capable (despite our mortality) of participating with a complementary other in the very same renewal of human possibility through procreation. Our genetic identity—manifest, for instance, in our distinctive appearance by which we are recognized by others and in our immune system by which we maintain our integrity against "foreign invasions"— also symbolizes and foreshadows exactly the unique, never-to-be-repeated character of each human life. In addition, human societies virtually everywhere have structured child-rearing responsibilities and systems of identity and relationships on the bases of these natural facts of begetting. Kinship is tied to origins, and identity, at least in part, is tied to kinship. It is against this background that we must consider the implications of clonal reproduction, and the alterations it might produce in how cloned children would regard themselves and how they would be regarded by others. What would cloning-to-produce-children mean for individual identity, for kinship, and for sense of self, not only for the cloned child but also for his or her family?

Unaided sexual procreation is an activity at once natural, private, mysterious, unmediated, unpredictable, and undesigned. With the arrival of techniques such as IVF to assist procreation in the face of infertility, the process becomes less private and more mediated. But although technique is used, the basic structure of sexual reproduction—the combination of genetic material from father and mother resulting in a genetically unique child—is unaltered, the outcome is still unpredictable, and the genetic endowment of the child remains uncontrolled and undesigned. Cloning-to-produce-children would seem to bring procreation under human control and direction. What would this mean? What are the implications of allowing reproductive activities to become increasingly technological and commercialized? Cloning would be the first instance in which parents could select in advance the precise (or nearly precise) genetic makeup of their child, by selecting the donor to be cloned. It therefore forces us to ask what might be the difference between begetting and making, to wonder whether cloning somehow crosses the line between them, and, if so, to consider whether and why that should worry us.

Though admittedly sketchy and incomplete, these preliminary reflections on the nature and meaning of human procreation should enable us to see cloning—and especially cloning-to-produce-children—in its most important human context and to understand its deepest implications for its practitioners and for society.

Cloning and Biomedical Science

Human procreation is not the only context for evaluating the prospect of human cloning. As a product of biotechnology, a potential means of assisted reproduction, and a possible source of cloned embryos for research and medical use, human cloning also points us to questions about the aims, ends, and means of biomedical science and technology. Ordinarily, we are not prompted to much reflection about what science is for and what goals technology should serve. Our society tacitly accepts the self-directing and self-augmenting character of these activities, and the vast majority of us support them because we esteem and benefit from their contributions to human understanding and human welfare. However, when developments such as cloning raise profound questions affecting fundamental moral values and social institutions, we are forced to consider the ends and means of science and technology, and to explore their standing in the scheme of human goods.

To provide a context for assessing human cloning and its possible benefits, we do well to remember the goals of medicine and modern science: the great value and importance of treating disease and relieving suffering, including the sorrows of infertility; and the great value and importance of gaining knowledge about the workings of nature, our own nature emphatically included. No one can doubt the merit of these noble aims. Yet there has always been some disagreement about the lengths to which we should allow ourselves to go in serving them. Questions therefore arise about the need for limits on scientific pursuits and technological activities, and, conversely, about the meaning of such limits for the scientific and technological enterprises.

To address these questions, we must appreciate the human good of biomedical science in its fullness, and we must ask about the necessary and sufficient conditions for its flourishing. We must recognize, among other things, the unpredictability of scientific discovery and technological innovation, and the importance, therefore, of keeping open lines of inquiry and experimentation regardless of current estimates of their likelihood of success. Although serendipity often favors the prepared mind, nature guards her secrets well, and even the best scientists are regularly surprised by where the keys to the locks are ultimately found.

But precisely because so much of biomedical science is exploratory and experimental, scientific inquiry is not just thought but also action, action often involving research on living subjects, including human beings. And precisely because the use of technologies often has unintended or undesirable side effects, affecting many human goods in addition to health, safety, and the relief of suffering, large questions are necessarily raised when the goods promoted by technology come into conflict with others. For example, is the need to discover new cures for the sick a moral imperative that should trump all other goods and values?

If not, then on what basis can it be limited? What moral boundaries should scientists and technologists respect as they continue their quests for knowledge and cures, whether or not they receive public funding? How can society establish and enforce such boundaries? And, on the other hand, how can science and technology be protected against unreasonable limitations imposed by excessively fearful legislators or overzealous regulators?

To be sure, these large questions are hard to answer in the abstract. As a result, they do not recommend themselves for much deliberation. Yet they are very close to the surface of the current debate about human cloning. Moreover, implicit answers to these questions, seldom articulated and rarely defended save by mere assertion, at least color and may even determine what people think should be done about human cloning. A clearer and more thoughtful awareness of the aims of biomedical science could help us assess whether and how human cloning might serve the ends of science and medicine and could help us more fully consider its possible benefits and potential drawbacks.

But we must consider not only the ends of science, but also the means it employs. Cloning, after all, is a technique, a means of reaching some desired end. Even if the purposes it might serve are worthy, it must still be evaluated as a means. Not every means employed in the pursuit of worthy ends can pass ethical muster. This truth is widely recognized in the establishment of canons of ethics regarding the use of human subjects in research. It is also recognized in the established practice of technology assessment, which seeks to find the least problematic and least dangerous means for achieving a desirable end.

For instance, as a means of treating infertility or of providing a suitable source of compatible organs for transplantation, cloning raises difficulties having to do with human dignity and the costs of "manufacture" of the sort discussed earlier. Human cloning also raises questions about the ethics of research with human subjects, with risks of harm to the child-to-be, the egg donor, and the woman who would bring the cloned child to birth, questions that we shall take up in some detail in Chapter Five. Yet the most highly controverted moral argument about human cloning research involves a human subject not always considered when the ethics of research is discussed: the early human embryo. Because all cloning begins with the production of embryonic clones, and because such clones are potentially highly useful in biomedical research, questions of the ethics of means are absolutely central to the debate about the morality of cloning.

Ethical questions regarding the use of human embryos in research are, of course, not unique to cloning. They have been central to the recent and continuing controversy about federal funding of research on human embryonic stem cells, because human embryos produced by IVF offer possibilities for medical advances, beyond their use in assisted reproduction. The use of embryos has aided research on early human development. These embryos are also the source of human embryonic stem cells, pluripotent cells* that may be induced to develop into all the tissues of the body. These stem cells thus may hold great promise for future treatment of chronic degenerative diseases and disabilities.

The difficulty arises because the embryos put to use in these ways are themselves destroyed. This fact raises serious and troubling questions about the proper way to regard these nascent human organisms and the morally appropriate way to treat them. Cloning techniques might provide an even more useful source of embryos for biomedical research than current IVF techniques. Human cloning could yield numerous identical embryos, could provide for the study of stem cells derived from individuals known to possess genetic diseases, and might eventually yield transplantable tissues for regenerative medicine that would escape immune rejection. Human cloning-for-biomedical-research therefore brings the moral question of means before us with even greater force. It calls on us to think of the good of medical advances and the relief of human suffering while at the same time considering our responsibilities to nascent human life and

---

* Pluripotent cells are those that can give rise to many different types of differentiated cells. See Glossary of Terms.

the possible harms to ourselves and future generations that may result from coming to regard the beginning stages of human life as raw material for use and exploitation.

While there is almost universal opposition to cloning-to-produce-children, the prospect of using cloned embryos in biomedical research has attracted significant support in the general public and among many scientists, patient advocacy groups, and policymakers. It therefore presents more complicated moral and policy challenges, and requires serious reflection on the duty of society to those of its members who are suffering, as well as its responsibility for nascent life. The precise character of both that duty and that responsibility is a subject of long-standing dispute, giving rise to a contentious but very important public debate.

Cloning and Public Policy

Beneath the current debate about human cloning lie major questions about the relation between science and technology and the larger society. Valuing freedom and innovation, our society allows scientists to inquire as they wish, to explore freely, and to develop techniques and technologies based on the knowledge they find, and on the whole we all benefit greatly as a result. We limit what scientists can do only in certain cases, as when their research requires the use of human subjects, in which case we erect rules and procedures to protect the health, safety, and dignity of the weak from possible encroachments by the strong. In more pervasive ways, we also shape what science does through public decisions about financial support and scientific education. With the uses of technology, we are sometimes more intrusive, establishing regulations to protect public health and safety or to preserve the environment. In rare cases, we even ban certain practices, such as the buying and selling of organs for transplantation. Yet, on the whole, the spirit of laissez-faire governs technological research, development, and use.

But when innovations arise that appear to challenge basic goods that we hold dear, or when the desirability of scientific and technological progress runs up against concerns for the protection of human life and well-being, we are forced to consider the tacit social contract between science and technology and the larger society. The current public and political deliberation about whether and how to restrict or prohibit human cloning forces us to do so in a most powerful way.

In addition, the current deliberation confronts us with the task of balancing important and commonly defended freedoms—the freedom of scientists to inquire, of technologists to invent, of individuals to reproduce, of entrepreneurs to invest and to profit—with the well-being of our society and its members. Circumstances in which otherwise beneficent freedoms can endanger paramount moral and social goods present serious challenges for free societies, and the prospect of cloning presents us with just such a challenge.

This is not an altogether unfamiliar challenge. There are other circumstances in which the freedom to explore, inquire, research, and develop technologies has been constrained. Biomedical science, as we have said, is restricted in its use of human subjects for research, and scientists are required to obtain informed consent and take great care to secure research subjects from harm. Scientific work is also restricted from activities that might harm the health of the general public, and from producing products that may endanger consumers. For example, the federal Food and Drug Administration sits at the juncture between development and marketing of medical products, regulating their introduction and use according to criteria of safety and efficacy. Our society has come to a near-total agreement on the need for such an agency and the importance of its work.

Human cloning, however, does not easily fall into any of the familiar classes of our experience with science. Nor do the ethical challenges it raises fit neatly into the categories of risks to health and safety that are ordinarily the basis of public oversight of science and technology. Raising ethical questions about ends as well as means, cloning is at once a potential human experiment, a possible aid to reproduction, an altogether new sort of procreative technique, a prospective means of human design, and a source of embryos and embryonic stem cells for research. It points back to familiar dilemmas of bioethics—including the ethics of human experimentation and embryo research—and it points forward to the sorts of challenges that will face us as biology gains greater technical prowess. It therefore invites us to think anew about the relationship between society and biomedical science and to evaluate the sufficiency of current institutions and practices that govern that relationship.

The potential dangers we face do not result from ill intent or bad faith. Neither of the prevailing caricatures in the cloning debate—the mad scientist on a blind quest for an inhuman immortality or the puritanical Luddite seeking to keep the future at bay—is accurate, appropriate, helpful, or fair. The challenge we face is not as easy as that. The challenge we face involves the conflict of competing sets of concerns and priorities, each in the service of vital human goods, and each driven by a desire to improve the human condition and to protect essential principles. The widely shared desire to cure disease, relieve suffering, understand human biology, and provide humankind with new and more powerful means of control can conflict, in this case, with the widely shared desire to respect life, individual identity, the dignity of human procreation, and other institutions and principles that keep our society healthy and strong. The challenge for our society is to determine, through public deliberation and thoughtful reflection, how best to adjudicate between these two desires and to determine what form to give to the tacit agreement between society and science, by which society promises freedom within bounds, and science affords us innovation, knowledge, and power while respecting reasonable limits.

The new and distinct challenges that confront us through cloning call upon us to consider the character of that tacit agreement, and to determine whether, and in what way, it might need to be amended and supplemented, especially in the face of the rapidly arriving new biomedical technologies that touch so directly upon our humanity. It is our hope in this report to contribute to just such a thoughtful consideration of the question.

The Report

In Chapter Two we present a brief history of human cloning. We summarize the scientific developments, the various public and political debates, and the actions of earlier panels and government bodies.

In Chapter Three we discuss the terminology of the cloning debate. We analyze the controversy over cloning terms, state the terms we intend to use, and lay out the rationale behind our choice of terms.

In Chapter Four we present a survey of the scientific aspects of human and animal cloning. We attempt to clarify what cloning is, where the science stands, and where it may be going.

In Chapter Five we discuss the ethical arguments for and against human cloning-to-produce-children. We consider reasons to create cloned children, concerns over safety and consent, and a series of moral objections.

In Chapter Six we discuss the ethical arguments for and against cloning-for-biomedical-research. We consider the likely medical benefits, the potential social and ethical difficulties, and the concern over the treatment of human embryos.

In Chapter Seven we discuss the public policy alternatives. We consider various options for government action, and present arguments for and against each.

In Chapter Eight, we present the Council's conclusions and offer our recommendations.

Chapter Two

Historical Aspects of Cloning

The previous chapter located human cloning in its larger human context. This chapter provides a brief history of human cloning, both as a scientific matter and as a subject of public discussion, debate, and legislation.[1] Although we present only selected highlights, rather than a comprehensive account, we seek to enable the reader to place the present debate about cloning and this report into their proper historical setting. Until recently, all discussion of human cloning concentrated exclusively on the prospect of clonal reproduction, the production of individuals genetically virtually identical to previously existing ones. Our historical account here reflects that emphasis. Yet we will also consider the emerging interest in cloning-for-biomedical-research, a prospect connected to the recent isolation of embryonic stem cells and their potential for the understanding and treatment of human disease and disability.

Scientific Milestones

As a scientific and technical possibility, human cloning has emerged as an outgrowth of discoveries or innovations in developmental biology, genetics, assisted reproductive technologies, animal breeding, and, most recently, research on embryonic stem cells. Assisted reproductive techniques in humans accomplished the in vitro fertilization of a human egg, yielding a zygote and developing embryo that could be successfully implanted into a woman's uterus to give rise to a live-born child. Animal breeders developed and refined these techniques with a view to perpetuating particularly valuable animals and maintaining laboriously identified genomes. Most recently, the isolation of embryonic stem cells and their subsequent in vitro differentiation into many different cell types have opened up possibilities for repairing and replacing diseased or nonfunctioning tissue, and thus possible research uses for cloned human embryos.

The German embryologist Hans Spemann conducted what many consider to be the earliest "cloning" experiments on animals. Spemann was interested in answering a fundamental question of biological development: does each differentiated cell retain the full complement of genetic information present initially in the zygote? In the late 1920s, he tied off part of a cell containing the nucleus from a salamander embryo at the sixteen-cell stage and allowed the single cell to divide, showing that the nucleus of that early embryo could, in effect, "start over." In a 1938 book, *Embryonic Development and Induction*, Spemann wondered whether more completely differentiated cells had the same capacity and speculated about the possibility of transferring the nucleus from a differentiated cell—taken from either a later-stage embryo or an adult organism—into an enucleated egg. As he explained it: "Decisive information about this question may perhaps be afforded by an experiment which appears, at first sight, to be somewhat fantastical. This experiment might possibly show that even nuclei of differentiated cells can initiate normal development in the egg protoplasms."[2] But Spemann did not know how to conduct such an experiment.

Research with frogs fourteen years later encouraged progress toward the "fantastical experiment." In 1952, the American embryologists Robert Briggs and Thomas J. King first successfully transferred nuclei from early embryonic cells of leopard frogs to enucleated leopard frog eggs. The "activated egg" began to divide and develop, became a multicellular embryo, and then became a tadpole.[3] Embryologists in other laboratories successfully repeated these initial experiments on different species of frogs. But additional experience also showed that the older and more differentiated a donor cell becomes, the less likely it is that its nucleus would be able to direct development.

In 1962, the British developmental biologist John Gurdon reported that he had produced sexually mature frogs by transferring nuclei from intestinal cells of tadpoles into enucleated frog eggs.[4]   The experiments had a low success rate and remained controversial. Gurdon continued this work in the 1970s, and he was able to produce tadpoles by transferring the nucleus of adult frog skin cells into enucleated frog eggs. Later experiments established that many factors in addition to the intact nucleus are crucial to success (see Chapter Four for further discussion). In retrospect, it is surprising that any of these earlier experiments produced positive results.[5] But despite their low success rates, these experiments demonstrated that the nucleus retained its full complement of genetic information and encouraged later investigators to explore mammalian cloning.

The birth of Louise Brown in 1978, the first baby conceived through in vitro fertilization (IVF), was also an important milestone, because it demonstrated that human birth was possible from eggs that were fertilized outside the body and then implanted into the womb. As for the possibility of cloning animals from adult cells—especially mammals—the work in the intervening years focused largely on the reprogramming of gene expression in somatic cells, the transfer of nuclei taken from embryos in mammals (beginning with mice in the 1980s), and finally the work of Ian Wilmut and his colleagues at the Roslin Institute with adult nuclei, which led to the birth of Dolly on July 5, 1996. Since then, similar success has been achieved in cloning other mammalian species, including cattle, goats, pigs, mice, cats, and rabbits (see Chapter Four).

The animal cloners did not set out to develop techniques for cloning humans. Wilmut's goal was to replicate or perpetuate animals carrying a valuable genome (for example, sheep that had been genetically modified to produce medically valuable proteins in their milk). Others, such as the cloners of the kitten CC, were interested in commercial ventures for the cloning of pets.[6] Yet the techniques developed in animals have encouraged a small number of infertility therapists to contemplate and explore efforts to clone human children. And, following the announcement in 1998 by James Thomson and his associates of their isolation of human embryonic stem cells, there emerged an interest in cloned human embryos, not for reproductive uses but as a powerful tool for research into the nature and treatment of human disease.

Human Cloning from Popular Literature to Public Policy: From **Brave New World** *to the Birth of Dolly*

Technological novelties are often imagined and discussed in literature, especially in science fiction, before they are likely or even possible in practice. This has certainly been the case with human cloning, whose place in the popular imagination precedes the earliest successful animal cloning experiments. Perhaps the most famous early modern account of human cloning is Aldous Huxley's *Brave New World* (1932), where natural human procreation has become a thing of the past, and where babies are produced in identical batches through "Bokanovsky's Process." As the novelist tells it:

> One egg, one embryo, one adult—normality. But a bokanovskified egg will bud, will proliferate, will divide . . . becoming anywhere from eight to ninety-six embryos—a prodigious improvement, you will agree, on nature. Identical twins—but not in piddling twos and threes . . . Standard men and women; in uniform batches.[7]

The relevance or irrelevance of Huxley's vision to the dilemmas of the present is of course a matter of serious disagreement. Some believe that fears of a "Brave New World" are fantasy divorced from both the political realities of modern liberal democracy and the facts of science. Others believe the book remains a prescient warning of where biological self-manipulation could take us—which is to say, to a world where family is obsolete, life is engineered to order in the laboratory, and human beings have reduced themselves to well-satisfied human animals.

In the late 1960s, following John Gurdon's successful cloning experiments, a more focused debate on both the likelihood and the ethical and social implications of human cloning began among scientists, theologians, and ethicists. At this time, the still hypothetical possibility of cloning humans was considered as a part of a broader eugenic project to improve the genetic stock of humans as a species. In a famous article published in *The American Naturalist* in 1966, entitled "Experimental Genetics and Human Evolution," Nobel laureate biologist Joshua Lederberg described what he took to be the prospects of "clonal reproduction." "Experimentally," he wrote, "we know of successful nuclear transplantation from diploid somatic as well as germline cells into enucleated amphibian eggs. There is nothing to suggest any particular difficulty about accomplishing this in mammals or man, though it will rightly be admired as a technical tour-de-force when it is first implemented." He also predicted "there will be little delay between demonstration and use."[8]

While Lederberg concluded his essay by exhorting his readers not to "mistake comment for advocacy," he clearly believed that clonal reproduction might offer a number of human benefits or improvements. "If a superior individual (and presumably then genotype) is identified, why not copy it directly, rather than suffer all the risks of recombinational disruption, including those of sex," he asked. "The same solace is accorded the carrier of genetic disease: why not be sure of an exact copy of yourself rather than risk a homozygous segregant;[*] or at worst copy your spouse and allow some degree of biological parenthood." He described other possibilities—such as "the free exchange of organ transplants with no concern for graft rejection" and more efficient communication between individuals in "stressed occupations."[9]

---

[*] *Homozygous segregant*: an individual carrying two copies of the same mutant gene, one inherited from each parent, and thus destined to suffer from a genetic disease.

In the end, Lederberg argued that "tempered clonality"—a mix of clonal and sexual reproduction—might, at least from a biological standpoint, "allow the best of both worlds—we would at least enjoy being able to observe the experiment of discovering whether a second Einstein would outdo the first one." Nevertheless, he acknowledged the possibility for "social frictions" and ethical dilemmas that might result from clonal reproduction—including whether "anyone could conscientiously risk the crucial experiment, the first attempt to clone a man." He suggested that the "mingling of individual human chromosomes with other mammals assures a gradualistic enlargement of the field and lowers the threshold of optimism or arrogance, particularly if cloning in other mammals gives incompletely predictable results." And he feared that social policy might become based on "the accidents of the first advertised examples" rather than "well-debated principles."[10]

In 1970, the theologian and ethicist Paul Ramsey responded to Lederberg's portrait of human cloning—and, more generally, to the prospects for human self-modification—in a book called *Fabricated Man: The Ethics of Genetic Control*. He argued that human cloning would violate the ethical responsibilities of both science and parenthood: it would involve experiments on the child-to-be; it would transform parenthood into manufacture; and it would burden children with the genetic predisposition of their "maker" and so deny the cloned child a unique independence in the very act of bringing him or her to life. "[T]o attempt to soar so high above an eminently human parenthood," Ramsey wrote, "is inevitably to fall far below—into a vast technological alienation of man …. The entire rationalization of procreation—its replacement by replication—can only mean the abolition of man's embodied personhood."[11]

Ramsey believed that such a willingness to experiment on human life—or to create sub-humans—showed how the effort to perfect and improve humankind through genetic control leads in fact to ethical coarsening and to a disregard for actual human beings. "In the present age," he wrote, "the attempt will be made to deprive us of our wits by comparing objections to schemes of progressive genetic engineering or cloning men to earlier opposition to inoculations, blood transfusions, or the control of malaria. These things are by no means to be compared: the practice of medicine in the service of life is one thing; man's unlimited self-modification of the genetic conditions of life would be quite another matter."[12]

The debate over human cloning and genetic manipulation continued in the early 1970s. The Nobel laureate geneticist James D. Watson testified before Congress in 1971 on the subject of human cloning. He described the science that was taking us there, including John Gurdon's success in cloning frogs and the work of R. G. Edwards and P. S. Steptoe "in working out the conditions for routine test-tube conception of human eggs."[13] "Human embryological development," Watson observed, "need no longer be a process shrouded in secrecy. It can become instead an event wide-open to a variety of experimental manipulations." Watson called for the creation of national and international committees to promote "wide-ranging discussion … at the informal as well as formal legislative level, about the manifold problems which are bound to arise if test-tube conception becomes a common occurrence."[14] "This is a decision not for the scientists at all," he said. "It is a decision of the general public—do you want this or not?" and something that "if we do not think about it now, the possibility of our having a free choice will one day suddenly be gone."[15]

In 1972, Willard Gaylin, a psychiatrist and co-founder of the newly formed Institute of Society, Ethics, and the Life Sciences (later called the Hastings Center), made James Watson's warnings about cloning even more dramatic—with a *New York Times Magazine* article titled "The Frankenstein Myth Becomes a Reality—We Have the Awful Knowledge to Make Exact Copies of Human Beings." Gaylin hoped that the prospect of human cloning would awaken the public—and the scientific community—to the larger ethical implications of the life sciences.[16] The same year, biologist and ethicist Leon R. Kass published an essay in *The Public Interest* called "Making Babies—The New Biology and the 'Old' Morality," which addressed the prospect of both in vitro fertilization and human cloning, and wondered whether "by tampering with and confounding [our] origins, we are involved in nothing less than creating a new conception of what it means to be human."[17]

In stark contrast to Gaylin and Kass, ethicist Joseph Fletcher argued that human cloning would not be dehumanizing at all, but would, in a number of circumstances, serve the good of both society and individuals. In his 1974 book *The Ethics of Genetic Control: Ending Reproductive Roulette*, he argued that "Good reasons in general for cloning are that it avoids genetic diseases, bypasses sterility, predetermines an individual's gender, and preserves family likenesses. It wastes time to argue over whether we should do it or not; the real moral question is when and why."[18] For Fletcher—unlike Ramsey, Gaylin, and Kass—genetic control would serve the human end of self-mastery and self-improvement, it would improve the quality of life for individuals, and it would aid the progress of the human species. Gunther Stent, a molecular biologist at the University of California at Berkeley, echoed this view that human cloning would contribute to human perfection. As he wrote in a 1974 article in *Nature*: "To oppose human cloning . . . is to betray the Western dream of the City of God. All utopian visionaries, from Thomas More to Karl Marx, think of their perfect societies as being populated not by men but by angels that embody all of the best and none of the worst human attributes."[19] With cloning, he suggested, such a city might one day be possible.

For several years, cloning remained a topic for fiction and philosophy, but fantasy had yet to turn into fact. In 1978, in a book titled *In His Image: The Cloning of a Man*, science writer David Rorvik claimed that he was involved in a secret project to clone a millionaire in Montana named "Max."[20] The book caused a flurry of reaction—ranging from horror to amusement to nearly universal skepticism and denunciation in the scientific community—and eventually led to hearings before Congress on May 31, 1978. Robert Briggs, who with Thomas King cloned the first frog embryo from blastula frog cells in 1952, declared that the work in frogs demonstrated not that human cloning is now or imminently possible, but that "cloning in man or any other animal is not just a technical problem to be solved soon but may, in fact, never occur."[21] James Watson, who just a few years earlier had urged a national conversation and possible legislation on human cloning because of the rapid advances in the science, declared that we would "certainly not [see the cloning of a man] in any of our lifetimes. I wouldn't be able to predict when we might see the cloning of a mouse, much less a man."[22] Rorvik eventually admitted that the book was a hoax.

In the years that followed, claims and counter-claims of scientific advances in mammalian cloning—including the controversy beginning in 1981 over whether any of several independent laboratories had actually cloned mice—prompted more public reaction and discussion about the issue. But there was no sustained or widespread public interest, and cloning lost its prominent place within the bioethics literature. The President's Bioethics Commission, in its 1982 report *Splicing Life,* briefly discussed human cloning as well as IVF, but held that both were beyond the scope of that report because they could be considered reproductive technologies that did not necessarily involve modifying the genome (pp. 9-10). With regard to human cloning in particular, the report added that the possibility had received a good deal of public attention and it was therefore important to emphasize that even if it ever did become possible in humans, it would not result in an identical being.[23]

The National Institutes of Health Human Embryo Research Panel, which issued a report in 1994 on federal funding for research involving preimplantation human embryos, deemed research involving nuclear transplantation, without transfer of the resulting cloned embryo to a uterus, as one type of research that was acceptable for federal support. The report noted that the majority on this point was narrow, with nearly as many panel members concluding that the ethical implications of nuclear transplantation should be studied further before any such research could be acceptable for federal funding (Exec. Summ., p. xvii). In its discussion of cloning techniques, the panel noted that many different procedures are all called "cloning," and said in a footnote, "Popular notions of cloning derive from science fiction books and films that have more to do with cultural fantasies than actual scientific experiments."[24]

Of course, there had been, in the meantime, continued scientific work in nuclear transplantation in animals—including mammals. And with the 1997 announcement of the cloning of Dolly, the prospect of human cloning once again became a prominent issue in public discussion, debate, and public life.

The Human Cloning Debate: From Dolly to the Present

In late February 1997, Ian Wilmut and his team at the Roslin Institute in Scotland announced that they had, by means of somatic cell nuclear transfer, successfully cloned the first mammal from an adult somatic cell—Dolly the sheep. President Bill Clinton and British Prime Minister Tony Blair immediately denounced any attempts to clone a human being, and the President asked his National Bioethics Advisory Commission (NBAC) to report within ninety days on the scientific, ethical, and legal questions surrounding the prospect of human cloning. Congress likewise held a series of hearings—the first one on March 12, 1997. A widespread—though not universal—consensus emerged that attempts to clone a human being would at present be irresponsible and immoral. As Wilmut explained before Congress, "Our own experiments to clone sheep from adult mammary cells required us to produce 277 'reconstructed' embryos. Of these, twenty-nine were implanted into recipient ewes, and only one developed into a live lamb. In previous work with cells from embryos, three out of five lambs died soon after birth and showed developmental abnormalities. Similar experiments with humans would be totally unacceptable."[25]

Most ethicists agreed, though for different reasons. All agreed that cloning attempts on human beings "at this time" would be reckless experiments on the child-to-be and therefore totally unjustified. Many stressed, as Ramsey, Gaylin, and Kass had done in the 1970s, that human cloning would undermine the human meaning of parenthood and identity; that it would mean a giant step toward genetic engineering, creating the first children whose genetic predisposition was known and selected in advance; and that it would turn procreation increasingly into a form of manufacture.[26] In contrast, some bioethicists, including John Robertson and Ruth Macklin, believed that human cloning presented no inherent threat to public or private morality, that government had no legal authority or justification for banning clonal reproduction, and that it must be judged in terms of its particular uses, not dismissed outright.[27]

In June 1997, NBAC released its report *Cloning Human Beings*, which concluded that

> At present, the use of this technique to create a child would be a premature experiment that would expose the fetus and the developing child to unacceptable risks. This in itself might be sufficient to justify a prohibition on cloning human beings at this time, even if such efforts were to be characterized as the exercise of a fundamental right to attempt to procreate.[28]

NBAC also pointed to other moral concerns "beyond the issue of the safety of the procedure," including "the potential psychological harms to children and effects on the moral, religious, and cultural values of society" that "merit further discussion." NBAC recommended a three-to-five-year federal moratorium on human cloning—stating that the consensus came from the fact that the technique was not yet safe—to be revisited and reevaluated after that time. "Whether upon such further deliberation our nation will conclude that the use of cloning techniques to create children should be allowed or permanently banned is, for the moment, an open question."[29]

In early 1998, the United States Senate considered legislation, proposed by Republican Senators Christopher Bond of Missouri, Bill Frist of Tennessee, and Judd Gregg of New Hampshire, to ban all human cloning permanently. Nearly all senators denounced clonal reproduction, but many believed that the proposed ban, which would have made it illegal to create human embryos by means of somatic cell nuclear transfer, would undermine potentially valuable scientific research. Democratic Senators Edward Kennedy of Massachusetts and Tom Harkin of Iowa led the opposition, with the widespread support of patient advocacy groups, scientific and medical organizations, and the biotechnology industry. As Senator Kennedy put it:

> Every scientist in America understands the threat this legislation poses to critical medical research. Every American should understand it, too. . . . Congress can and should act to ban cloning of human beings during this session. But it should not act in haste, and it should not pass legislation that goes far beyond what the American people want or what the scientific and medical community understands is necessary or appropriate.[30]

The legislation died after heated debate, and the concern over human cloning temporarily lost urgency and subsided.

In November 1998, a new scientific discovery was unveiled that would soon provoke a different public policy debate, one that would become entangled with the ethical and social questions surrounding human cloning. James Thomson and John Gearhart separately announced the isolation of human embryonic stem cells—multipotent cells (see Glossary of Terms) derived from human embryos that they believed hold great promise for curing or treating many diseases and injuries. The discovery led to another wave of hearings on, and interest in, the ethics of biological science. It also renewed debate over whether embryo research should be eligible for public funding (since 1996, Congress had prohibited federal funding of research involving the destruction of human embryos). One subject under consideration was the possible future use of cloned human embryos for stem cell research, which some scientists believed might be uniquely useful for understanding embryological development and genetic disease and for possible use in stem cell therapies.

In August 2000—after another NBAC study—President Clinton announced new guidelines that would have altered the ban on federal funding of embryo research. The new guidelines, proposed by the National Institutes of Health, stipulated that the agency would fund research on embryonic stem cells so long as public funds were not used to destroy the embryos, the embryos were left over from IVF clinics, and donors of the embryos consented to the research.

In early 2001, President George W. Bush announced that he would review these guidelines rather than implement them immediately.* Around the same time, a number of pro-cloning groups and fertility doctors—including the Raelians, who believe that humans are the products of cloning by aliens—announced their intention to clone human beings by the end of the year. Other individuals and scientific organizations worked to protect possible cloning research from future restrictions, though some scientists (such as Rudolf Jaenisch and Ian Wilmut[31]) publicly argued against cloning-to-produce-children. A flurry of hearings on human cloning soon followed—the first one in the House of Representatives on March 28, 2001, and continuing in both the House and the Senate throughout the summer. The hearings addressed cloning-to-produce-children as well as issues related to cloning-for-biomedical-research.

Two general approaches to banning human cloning emerged. The first approach, proposed in a bill sponsored by Republican Representative David Weldon of Florida and Democratic Representative Bart Stupak of Michigan in the House, and Republican Senator Sam Brownback of Kansas and Democratic Senator Mary Landrieu of Louisiana in the Senate, called for a ban on all human cloning, including the creation of cloned embryos for

---

* On August 9, 2001, President Bush announced his new policy: federal funding would be made available for research using only those human embryonic stem cell lines that were already in existence (that is, lines that had been derived prior to that date).

biomedical research. The second approach, proposed in a bill sponsored by Republican Senators Arlen Specter of Pennsylvania and Orrin Hatch of Utah and Democratic Senators Diane Feinstein of California and Edward Kennedy of Massachusetts, sought to prohibit human reproductive cloning, while allowing the use of cloning technology to produce stem cells, by making it illegal to implant or attempt to implant cloned human embryos "into a uterus or the functional equivalent of a uterus."

On July 31, 2001, the House of Representatives passed the Weldon-Stupak bill (the ban on all human cloning) by a vote of 265 to 162. In November 2001, scientists at Advanced Cell Technology, Inc., of Worcester, Massachusetts, one of the leading commercial advocates of cloning-for-biomedical-research, reported what they claimed were the first cloned human embryos. The announcement—along with continued debate on the possible use of cloned human embryos for stem cell research—left the issue in the United States Senate, where it stands as of this writing.

Meanwhile, the general public has consistently expressed the view that human cloning is wrong—most recently, a Gallup poll from May 2002 that showed opposition to cloning to produce a child at 90 percent, and opposition to "cloning of human embryos for use in medical research" at 61 percent. Asked about medical research using stem cells obtained from human embryos (with no mention of how the embryo was generated), 52 percent found it morally acceptable, while 51 percent found acceptable the "cloning of human cells from adults for use in medical research."[32]

In addition to activity at the federal level, many states have been active. As of this writing, twenty-two states have considered various policy alternatives on cloning, and six have passed legislation.*

* As of June 2002 three states (Iowa, Michigan, and Virginia) ban both cloning-to-produce-children and cloning-for-biomedical-research. Two states (Louisiana and Rhode Island) ban cloning-to-produce-children, but also have embryo-research laws that appear to prohibit cloning-for-biomedical-research.

Several nations, including Denmark, France, Norway, Spain, and Canada have passed or sought either partial or total bans. For example, in the United Kingdom, cloning-to-pro-duce-children is forbidden but cloned embryos up to fourteen days old may be used in biomedical research. In Germany, all human cloning is forbidden by law. There are also efforts now at the United Nations and other international organizations to pass a world-wide ban on human cloning—with many of the same disagreements internationally as there are nationally about what kind of ban to pass.

ENDNOTES

1 Since the birth of Dolly, several volumes on the history and significance of cloning have been published, including Kolata, G., *Clone: The Road to Dolly and the Path Ahead*, New York: Morrow and Company, 1998, and National Bioethics Advisory Commission [NBAC], *Cloning Human Beings*, Bethesda, MD: Government Printing Office, 1997. In addition, several valuable anthologies have been edited, including Kristol, W., and E. Cohen , *The Future is Now*, Lanham, MD: Rowman and Littlefield, 2002, and Nussbaum, M., and C.R. Sunstein, *Clones and Clones*, New York: Norton, 1998.

2 See Spemann, H., *Embryonic Development and Induction* (New Haven, CT: Yale University Press, 1938). As quoted in Kolata, G., *Clone: The Road to Dolly and the Path Ahead* (New York: Morrow and Company, 1998), p. 61.

3 Briggs, R., and T. J. King, "Transplantation of living nuclei from blastula cells into enucleated frog's eggs," *Proceedings of the National Academy of Sciences* (USA) 38: 455-463, 1952.

4 Gurdon, J. B., "The developmental capacity of nuclei taken from intestinal epithelium cells of feeding tadpoles," *Journal of Embryology and Experimental Morphology* 10, 622-640, 1962.

5 A fact also noted by NBAC in *Cloning Human Beings,* p. 18.

One state (California) has banned cloning-to-produce-children, until Dec. 31, 2002, but has no embryo-research law and thus effectively permits cloning-for-biomedical-research.

6 Regalado, A., "Only Nine Lives for Kitty? Not if She Is Cloned," *Wall Street Journal*, February 14, 2002, p. B1. Kluger, J., "Here Kitty Kitty!" *Time*, February 17, 2002.

7 Huxley, Aldous., *Brave New World* (New York: Harper Perennial, 1998), p. 6-7. Originally published by Harper & Brothers, 1932.

8 Lederberg, J., "Experimental Genetics and Human Evolution," *The American Naturalist*, September-October 1966, Vol. 100, No. 915, pp. 527.

9 Ibid, p. 531, 527, 528.

10 Ibid, p. 528, 529, 531.

11 Ramsey, P., *Fabricated Man: The Ethics of Genetic Control* (New Haven, CT: Yale University Press, 1970), p. 89.

12 Ibid, p. 95.

13 Watson, J., "Moving Toward the Clonal Man," *The Atlantic Monthly*, May 1971, p. 51. (This article is a slightly modified version of Watson's congressional testimony.)

14 Ibid, p. 51, 53.

15 Proceedings before the Committee on Science and Astronautics, U. S. House of Representatives, Ninety-Second Congress, January 26, 27, and 28, 1971, p. 344.

16 Gaylin, W., "The Frankenstein Myth Becomes a Reality—We Have the Awful Knowledge to Make Exact Copies of Human Beings," *The New York Times Magazine*, March 5, 1972, p. 12ff.

17 Kass, L., "Making Babies—the New Biology and the 'Old' Morality," *The Public Interest*, Winter 1972, Number 26, p. 23.

18 Fletcher, J., *The Ethics of Genetic Control: Ending Reproductive Roulette* (New York: Anchor Books, 1974), p. 154.

19 Stent, G., "Molecular Biology and Metaphysics," *Nature*, Vol. 248, No. 5451, April 26, 1974, p. 781. As quoted in Kolata op. cit., p. 92.

20 Rorvik, D. M., *In His Image: The Cloning of a Man* (New York: J. B. Lippincott, 1978).

21 As quoted in Kolata, op. cit., p. 103.

22 Interview by C. P. Anderson, "In His Own Words: Nobel Laureate James Watson Calls Report of Cloning People 'Science Fiction Silliness,'" *People*, April 17, 1978, pp. 93-95. As quoted in Kolata, op. cit., p. 104.

23 President's Commission for the Study of Ethical Problems in Medicine and Biomedical and Behavioral Research, *Splicing Life: A Report on the Social and Ethical Issues of Genetic Engineering with Human Beings*, November 1982.

24 National Institutes of Health, Ad Hoc Group of Consultants to the Advisory Committee to the Director, *Report of the Human Embryo Research Panel*, September 1994, p. 28.

25 Hearing before the Subcommittee on Public Health and Safety of the Committee on Labor and Human Resources, United States Senate, March 12, 1997. p. 22.

26 See, for example, Kass, L., "The Wisdom of Repugnance," *The New Republic*, June 2, 1997, pp. 17-26, and "Preventing a Brave New World, *The New Republic*, May 21, 2001, pp. 30-39.

27 Robertson, J.A., "A Ban on Cloning and Cloning Research Is Unjustified," testimony before the National Bioethics Advisory Commission, March 14, 1997. Macklin, R., testimony before NBAC, March 14, 1997.

28 NBAC, *Cloning Human Beings*, 1997, pp. ii-iii.

29 Ibid, p. iii.

30 *Congressional Record*, February 9, 1998, pp. S513-514.

31 Jaenisch, R., and I. Wilmut, "Don't clone humans!" *Science* 291: 5513, March 30, 2001.

32 Saad, L. "Cloning Humans Is a Turn-Off to Most Americans" *Gallup Poll Analyses*, May 16, 2002.

Chapter Three

On Terminology

We begin our presentation of the important matter of terminology by listing the crucial terms used in this report:

- *Human cloning.*
- *Cloning-to-produce-children.*
- *Cloning-for-biomedical-research.*
- *Cloned human embryo.*

The rest of this chapter will develop the meaning of these terms and provide the analysis and argumentation that have led us to these choices. Because there is much to be learned about the subject through the discussion of alternative terminologies, and because we believe strongly that the judicious use of language is necessary for sound moral choice, we present our discussion of this matter at some length.

Introduction: The Importance of Careful Use of Names

Fruitful discussion of the ethical and policy issues raised by the prospects of human cloning—as with any other matter—can proceed only if we can find appropriate and agreed-upon terms for describing the processes and products involved. Before we can get to possible moral or policy arguments or disagreements, we need to agree about what to call that about which we are arguing. As a contribution to public understanding, we emphasize that this is not an easy thing to do, and we indicate how and why we have gone about making our terminological choices.

What exactly is meant by the term "cloning"? What criterion justifies naming an entity a "clone"? How is the term "cloning" related to what scientists call "somatic cell nuclear transfer (SCNT)" or "nuclear transplantation"? What should we call the single-cell entity that results from SCNT, and what should we call it once it starts to divide and develop? How, if at all, should our names for such activities or such entities be affected by the purposes we have for engaging in the activities or for using the entities?

As these questions imply, there is much confusion today about the terms used in discussing human cloning. There is honest disagreement about what names should be used, and there are also attempts to select and use terms in order to gain advantage for a particular moral or policy position. One difficulty is the difference between the perspective of science and the perspective of lived human experience. People who look at the phenomena of human reproduction and development through the lens of science will see and describe things in terms that often differ widely from those in ordinary usage; moreover, when an ordinary term is used in scientific parlance, it sometimes is given a different meaning. Similar divergences are possible also for people who look at these matters through the lens of different cultural, philosophical, or religious beliefs. Yet at the same time, all of us—scientists or not, believers or not—encounter these same matters on the plane of lived human experience, for which the terms of everyday speech may well be more suitable. Because this same common (nonscientific) discourse is also the medium of discourse for the ethical and policy discussions, we shall strive to stay close to common speech, while at the same time making the best use we can of scientific findings to avoid mistakes and misconceptions.

Advisers to decision makers should strive not only for accuracy, but also for fairness, especially because the choice of names can decisively affect the way questions are posed and, hence, how answers are given. The issue is not a matter of semantics; it is a matter of trying fairly to call things by names that correctly describe them, of trying to fit speech to fact as best one can. For the sake of clarity, we should at least stipulate clearly the meanings we intend by our use of terms. But we should also try to choose terms that most accurately convey the descriptive reality of the matter at hand. If this is well done, the moral arguments can then proceed on the merits, without distortion by linguistic sloppiness or chicanery.

Many of the terms that appear in the debate about cloning are confusing or are used in a confused manner.

First, there are difficulties concerning the terms that seek to name the *activity* or *activities* involved: cloning, asexual reproduction, reproductive cloning, nonreproductive cloning, research cloning, therapeutic cloning, somatic cell nuclear transfer (or nuclear transplantation), nuclear transfer for stem cell research, nuclear transplantation to produce stem cells, nuclear transfer for regenerative medicine. At stake are such questions as whether all acts of SCNT should be called cloning. Some worry that the term "cloning" unfairly prejudices people against the activity when it is used to describe research activities.

Second, there are difficulties concerning the terms that seek to name the *entity* or *entities* that result from human cloning (or human SCNT): cell, egg, activated cell, totipotent cell, clonote, reconstituted (or reconstructed) egg, zygote, clump of cells, embryo, human embryo, human organism, blastocyst, clonocyst, potential human being, human being, human clone, person. At stake here is the nature—and the possible *moral* status—of the entities that are involved in the subsequent manipulations, whether for producing a child or for use in biomedical research. Some worry that use of any term but "embryo" will unfairly prejudice people in favor of embryo-destructive activities by hiding from view the full import of the activity.

Third, there are difficulties concerning the terms that seek to describe the *relation* between the cloned entity and the person whose somatic cell nucleus was transferred to produce the cloned entity: genetic copy, replica, genetically virtually identical, noncontemporary twin, delayed genetic twin, clone.

Tools of Analysis

As a prelude to examining the *activity* or the *deed* of cloning, some general analytical observations will be helpful. Although all aspects of an activity or action are relevant to understanding its full human meaning, when describing a deed it is sometimes useful to distinguish *what* it is from both *how* it is done and *why* it is done. The act itself (*what*) may be accomplished by a variety of means or techniques (*how*), and it may be undertaken for a variety of motives or purposes (*why*). To be sure, there is a danger of distortion in this disaggregating analysis of human activity, and there is disagreement about the degree to which the motives or purposes of the agent are to be reckoned in the description of the act itself. People argue, for example, whether "mercy killing" differs *as an act* from murdering a rival (or executing a murderer or killing someone in self-defense), or whether they are all equally acts of homicide (literally, "killing a human being") whose *moral* meaning ("Is it justified or not?" "Is it wrong or not?") we can then proceed to debate, if we wish, by attending not only to the bare act of taking a human life but also to the agent's motive and purpose. Though we do not wish to beg this question, the very existence of this disagreement suggests that we do well not to ignore the naked act itself, for it may have a meaning independent of what moved the agent, a meaning relevant to subsequent moral assessment that we do not wish to overlook.

To illustrate: in vitro fertilization (IVF: the merging of egg and sperm outside the human body [*in vitro* = "in glass"], yielding a zygote that is the beginning stage of a new living being) is the deed (*what*). It is an act of "fertilization," of making fertile, of making the egg cell ready and able to develop into a human organism. This fertilization may be accomplished in at least two ways (*how*): by merely mixing egg and sperm, allowing the sperm to find and penetrate the egg, or by the technique of injecting individual sperm directly into the egg (a technique known as intracytoplasmic sperm injection, ICSI). And it may be done for the (proximate) purpose (*why*) of initiating a pregnancy, in turn for the (ultimate) purpose of providing a child for an infertile couple; or it may be done for the (proximate) purpose of providing living human embryos for basic research on normal and abnormal embryological development, in turn for the (ultimate) purposes of understanding human development or of discovering cures for diseases and producing tissues for regenerative medicine. Though the technique used or the purposes served may differ, in *one* crucial respect the deed (IVF) remains the same and bears a common *intrinsic meaning*: a human zygote, the first stage of a new human being, is intentionally produced outside the body and exists in human hands and subject to human manipulation.

As it happens, this fact is more or less accurately reflected in the descriptive terminology used for IVF. Interestingly enough, unlike the situation with cloning, no one distinguishes between "reproductive IVF" and "therapeutic IVF" or "research IVF," naming the activity or deed after the motive or purpose of the agent. This may reflect the historical fact that IVF was initiated by people who were interested in using it to produce live-born children for infertile couples; the research use of "surplus" embryos produced by IVF came only later. But it happens that this common name is also descriptively apt and remains so regardless of why IVF was done in a particular case: the deed *is* fertilization of egg by sperm, producing a living human zygote, the first stage of the development of a new human being.

It should be noted that, although we began by trying to describe the deed rather than the product of the deed, the two aspects merged necessarily. The meaning of the act of "fertilization" falls forward onto the nature of the "object" that fertilization produces: the fertilized egg or zygote or earliest embryo.* (By contrast, there

---

* A more careful analysis of the *what* of this activity would distinguish between the activity itself and the product that results from it. Unlike nonproductive activities, such as dancing ("How can we know the dancer from the dance?"), the work (activity) of making or producing results in separable objects or works (products). Although shoemaking completes itself in the production of a shoe, the shoe as *result* is distinct from the *activity* of shoemaking. Similarly, though fertilization is an activity that is intelligible only as issuing in a fertilized egg, the now-fertile egg as *result* or *product* stands apart from the deed of IVF. One reason that the word "fertilization" works so well in describing IVF

is nothing in the name of the technique "intracytoplasmic sperm injection" that even hints at the immediate result or goal of the intended injection.) Similar attention to the nature of the product may turn out to be indispensable for a proper characterization of the activity of cloning.

Cloning: Toward an Appropriate Terminology

Though much of the terminological confusion and controversy concerns the way to describe the different *kinds* of cloning practices that are envisioned, the term "cloning" itself is not without its own ambiguities. A "clone" (noun, from the Greek *klon*, "twig") refers to a *group* of genetically identical molecules, cells, or organisms descended from a single common ancestor, as well as to *any one* of the one or more individual organisms that have descended asexually from a common ancestor. Both the group and each of its members are "a clone." "To clone" (verb) is to duplicate or produce a genetic duplicate or duplicates of a molecule, cell, or individual organism. The replication of DNA fragments in the laboratory is called "DNA cloning." The physical isolation of a single cell and its subsequent multiplication in tissue culture into a population of descendants is referred to as "single cell cloning." The laboratory culture of bacteria and the asexual propagation of plants by means of cuttings are instances of organismal cloning. Cloning of higher organisms is more complex: all cloning of vertebrate organisms must begin at the embryonic stages. Contrary to what some people imagine, cloning of amphibians or mammals (including human beings) is not the direct duplication ("photocopying") of an adult organism.

In the sense relevant here, "cloning" is a form of asexual reproduction (parthenogenesis* is another), the production of a new in-

---

is that it is a very rich term, pointing both to cause and effect, backward to the deed and forward to the future prospects of the product.

* Parthenogenesis (see Glossary of Terms), the development of an organism directly from an unfertilized egg that has been artificially induced to undergo

dividual not by the chance union of egg and sperm but by some form of replication of the genetic makeup of a single existing or previously existing individual. (In biological or functional terms, the core of sexual reproduction is not bodily intercourse but the fusion of male and female *germ cells*; thus IVF, though it takes place outside the body, is—biologically speaking—a form of sexual reproduction.) Cloning is the activity of producing a clone, an individual or group of individuals genetically virtually identical to the precursor that is being "replicated."*

Cloning-to-Produce-Children; Cloning-for-Biomedical-Research

In much of the current public discussion, we encounter a distinction between two sorts of cloning: "reproductive" and "therapeutic." The distinction is based entirely on the differing goals of the cloners: in the first case, the goal is the production of a (cloned) child; in the second case, the development of treatments for diseases (suffered not by the clone, but by others). We recognize the

---

development, is, in principle, another method of asexual reproduction. Although parthenogenetic reproduction has been successfully achieved in amphibians, in mammalian species there are as yet no reports of live births following parthenogenesis. Thus, there is at present little reason to believe that live-born human beings can be produced via parthenogenesis. It is therefore not the subject of this report, although many of the things said about cloning via somatic cell nuclear transfer would be applicable to asexual reproduction through parthenogenesis.

* Although cloning, like fertilization, is responsible for bringing forth a new organism, the activities are named in very different ways, yet in each case emphasizing the fundamental intention of the activity. "Fertilization" describes the activity in terms of the capacitation of the egg, as a result of which development begins. "Cloning" describes the activity in terms of *the relation between the progenitor and the product*. In cloning by somatic cell nuclear transfer, the egg, though it is activated as if it were fertilized, is not cloned; cloned rather is the donor from whom the nucleus was taken, and the resulting organism (at all stages of development) is a clone of the donor. The name of the activity, "cloning," even more than "in vitro fertilization," refers to the *product* of the activity, an identical (or nearly identical) entity.

distinction and the need for terms to describe the difference. But the terms currently in vogue have their difficulties. Both terms have been criticized by partisans of several sides of the debate, and for understandable reasons.

Some object to the term "reproductive cloning" used as a term of distinction, because they argue that *all* cloning is reproductive. Their reason: all human cloning intends and issues in the production of a cloned human embryo, a being distinct from the components used to generate it, a new human being in the earliest stage of development or "reproduction." (This claim, we would suggest, is at this stage a descriptive point, not yet a normative one; *it does not necessarily imply that such a being is fully human or "one of us," hence deserving of the moral and social protection accorded "persons."*) The fact that only some of these embryonic cloned humans are wanted for baby-producing purposes does not, in the view of these critics, alter this fact about their being. In support of their claim that cloning occurs (only) at the beginning, they note that once the cloning act of nuclear transfer has occurred, all new influences that act upon the new human organism cease to be "genetic" (nature) and are now "environmental" (nurture). Instead of "reproductive cloning," we shall speak of "cloning-to-produce-children."

Others object to the term "therapeutic cloning" for related reasons. The act of cloning embryos may be undertaken with healing motives. But it is not *itself* an act of healing or therapy.[*] The beneficiaries of any such acts of cloning are, at the moment, hypothetical and in the future. And if medical treatments do eventually result, the embryonic clone from which the treatment was derived will not itself be the beneficiary of any therapy. On the contrary, this sort of cloning actually takes apart (or destroys) the embryonic being that results from the act of cloning.

---

[*] Compare, in this respect, what used to be called "therapeutic abortion," an abortion undertaken in cases in which pregnancy threatened the life of the pregnant woman and where abortion was therefore intended to save the woman's life. Similarly, we might call the removal of a cancerous kidney a "therapeutic nephrectomy"; we would never use the term to refer to the removal of a kidney for donation to another person in transplantation.

To avoid the misleading implications of calling any cloning "therapeutic," we prefer the terms "research cloning" or "cloning for research," which also more accurately indicate the purpose of the activity. Yet some may find fault with this replacement. Because it appears to be a deliberate substitution for "therapeutic cloning," it may seem to imply that the scientists have abandoned the pursuit of medical cure in favor of research as an end in itself. Believing that producing cloned embryos just for research would seem to be less justifiable than producing them with healing motives, these critics of the term "research cloning" want to avoid giving the impression that scientists want to experiment on new life just to satisfy their curiosity. We believe that this legitimate concern can be addressed by appending the adjective "biomedical" to make clear that the aim of the research is to seek cures and treatments for human diseases. We therefore opt to use the term "cloning-for-biomedical-research."

Some proponents of the activity called "therapeutic cloning" also now object to the term, but not because of the adjective. Though it was proponents who originally coined and used the term, some of them now want to shed the term "cloning," fearing that the bad or distressing connotations of the latter will weigh against the activity itself. Cloning, they insist, should be reserved for the activity that produces live-born cloned babies; it should not apply to the initial act that starts the process, which they would rather call "somatic cell nuclear transfer" or "nuclear transplantation."[1] The reason for such re-description is not wholly cosmetic and rhetorical; because the researchers are primarily interested in obtaining pluripotent* stem cells, their focus is on the somatic cell nucleus and what must be done to it (transfer or transplantation) in order for it to revert to the undifferentiated condition of the primordial stem cell stage. Nevertheless, such terminological substitution is problematic, for the following reasons.

---

* Pluripotent cells are those that can give rise to many different types of differentiated cells. See Glossary of Terms.

Although as a scientific matter "somatic cell nuclear transfer" or "nuclear transplantation" may accurately describe the *technique* that is used to produce the embryonic clone, these terms fail to convey the nature of the deed itself, and they hide its human significance. The deed, fully described, is the production of a living human entity (or "embryo" or "organism"; of the right name for the product, more later) that is genetically virtually identical to the donor organism, a fact or meaning not captured in the name for the technique or method, the transfer of a somatic cell nucleus (into an unfertilized egg whose own nucleus has been removed or inactivated).* As a name, SCNT is not a fully accurate description even of the technique itself. It makes no reference to the intended and direct result of the deed of nuclear transfer. It also omits mention of the fact that the recipient of the transferred nucleus is an (enucleated) *egg* cell (rather than another kind of cell), which then can be made to initiate cell division as if it were just like a zygote produced by fertilization. The further amendments, "somatic cell nuclear transfer *for stem cell research*" or "nuclear transplantation *for regenerative medicine*" or "nuclear transplantation *to produce stem cells*" only compound the difficulty, mixing in the purpose of the activity with its technique, thus further obscuring the immediate meaning of the act itself, the production of a living cloned human embryo.

Cloned Human Embryo: The Product of SCNT

What shall we call the product of SCNT? The technical description of the cloning method (that is, SCNT) omits all reference not only to cloning but also to the *immediate product* of the activity. This obscurity enables some to argue that the immediate product of SCNT is not an "embryo" but rather "an egg" or "an unfertilized egg" or "an activated cell," and that the subsequent stages of development should not be called embryos but "clumps of cells" or "activated cells." To be sure, there are genuine difficulties and perplexities regarding what names to use, for we are dealing with an entity new in our experience. Partly for this reason, some people recommend avoiding the effort to describe the nature of the prod-

---

* This reduction of an act to its mechanism is roughly analogous to describing walking as "sequential alternate leg advancement" (SALA).

uct, preferring instead to allow the *uses we human beings have for it* to define its being, and hence its worth. But, for reasons of both truth and ethical conduct, we reject this approach as improper. We are all too familiar with instances in which some human beings have defined downward the status of other beings precisely to exploit them with impunity and with a clear conscience. Thus, despite the acknowledged difficulties in coming to know it accurately, we insist on making the effort to describe the product of SCNT as accurately and as fairly as we can.

The initial product of SCNT is a single cell, but it is no ordinary cell. It is also an "egg" and a "reconstituted egg." But even that is not the whole story. The "reconstituted" egg is *more* than reconstituted; it has been capacitated for development. Because the egg now has a diploid nucleus, it has become something beyond what it was before: it now contains in a single nucleus the full complement of genetic material necessary for producing a new organism.* And being an *egg* cell, it uniquely offers the cytoplasmic environment that can support this development. The product of SCNT thus resembles and can be made to act like a fertilized egg, a cell that not only has the full complement of chromosomes but also is capable (in animals) or may be capable (in humans) of developing into a new organism. In other words, in terms of its future prospects, it is a "zygote-like entity" or a (cloned) "zygote equivalent."†

---

* The original egg had a haploid nucleus, containing only half the chromosomes necessary for development. The diploid nucleus contains the full amount. See Chapter Four.

† Technically, the term "zygote" (from a Greek root meaning "yoke") refers to the primordial cell that forms from the union of egg and sperm and the fusion (the yoking together) of their nuclei as the first step in the development of a new life that has come from the joining of its two parents. It is for this reason technically inappropriate to call the product of an asexual initiation a "zygote," though it may be its functional equivalent. The term "clonote" has been suggested as the strict analogue of "zygote," identifying the primordial cell formed in cloning by its special origin: just as a zygote arises from the "yoking together" of *two* elements, so a "clonote" arises from the act of clonal propagation from a *single*, already *existing* organism. (Similarly, the term "parthenote" for the primary product of parthenogenesis would accurately indicate that it arises from the "virgin" [unfertilized] egg alone; *parthenos*,

The initial product of SCNT is, to be sure, not just a cell but an *active* cell. (More precisely, it is a cell that can be activated by electric stimulation.) But "activated cell" is much too vague to describe the activity of which it is capable. For, once stimulated, the activity of this "cell" produced by SCNT is nothing other than human embryological development, initiated and directed by the cell itself. The processes of cellular growth, chromosomal replication, cell division, and (ultimately) differentiation into the tissues and organs of the organism are coordinated processes under the governance of the immanent developmental plan encoded in the cell's genetic material. In other words, the product of SCNT is an organism in its germinal stage, and its activities are those of an integrated and self-developing whole.*

Another suggested name, better than "activated cell," is "totipotent cell"—a cell that is "capable of all." But this too is ambiguous. If what is meant is that it can (and will, should it be stimulated to do so) become "any and all" of the different kinds of cells in the body, then it is an insufficient meaning. For, as explained in the previous paragraph, *this* totipotent cell may also become the "all" that is the integrated *whole* (cloned) mature organism itself (along with a portion of the placenta that would give it nourishment). In this second and fuller meaning of "totipotent," a totipotent cell is then just a *functional* synonym for the "zygote": "zygote" etymologically reminds one of the cell's origins in egg-joined-to-sperm; "totipotency" describes what it is capable of. A fertilized egg is precisely a "totipotent" cell; the product of human SCNT is, we assume, its equivalent.

Greek for "virgin.") The term "clonote" also has the merit of carrying the *clonal* character of the entity in its name.

* For the reasons given in this paragraph, we reject the suggestion that the immediate product of SCNT and the cells it gives rise to should be considered "cells in tissue culture." Unlike *somatic* cells grown in laboratory culture, the immediate product of SCNT, although (like cultured tissues) it grows in culture media outside the body, is the germ of a new *organism*, not merely of other cells just like itself.

In some discussions, the next few stages of the developing cloned human entity have been described as "clumps of cells." Yet, for reasons already given, this is only partially accurate. Viewed externally, under the microscope, the developing embryo will appear as two, then four, then eight cells "clumped" together, and the 100-to-200-cell blastocyst stage will indeed appear as a "ball of cells." Yet there is more here than meets the eye, for the "clump" is governed by an internal principle of development that shapes and directs its transformations. Thus, this ball or clump is not a mere heap or aggregate; it is a primordial and unfolding whole that functions as a whole and that is in the process of developing (or attempting to develop) into a mature whole being. Of course, if development is not pursued or not allowed to happen because of disruption, then the "clump of cells" description may be rendered accurate not just microscopically but also biologically. But as long as development continues and the developing entity is intact, that is not the case.

It would seem, then, that—whatever the reason for producing it—the initial product of somatic cell nuclear transfer is a living (one-celled) cloned human embryo. The *immediate* intention of transferring the nucleus is precisely to produce just such an entity: one that is alive (rather than nonliving), one that is human (rather than nonhuman or animal), and one that is an embryo, an entity capable of developing into an articulated organismic whole (rather than just a somatic cell capable only of replication into more of the same cell type). This is the intended primary product of performing SCNT, whether the ultimate motive or purpose is producing a live-born child from the cloned embryo or conducting scientific research on the cloned embryo. Also, the blastocyst stage that develops from this one-celled cloned embryo will be the same being, whether it is then transferred to a woman's uterus to begin a pregnancy or is used as a source of stem cells for research and possible therapy for others.

Yet, not surprisingly, objections have been raised to calling this cloned entity an "embryo," objections having to do both with its origins and with the uncertainty about the extent of its developmental potential. There are also objections having to do not with the facts but with public connotations and perceptions: for some members of the public, the word "embryos" apparently conjures images of miniature babies. If "nuclear transplantation to produce stem cells" seems to some people to be unfairly morally *neutered* terminology, "embryo" seems to other people to be unfairly morally *loaded* terminology, especially when used to describe an entity barely visible to the naked eye. We acknowledge this problem and recognize that, despite our best efforts, such difficulties in public perception probably cannot be simply corrected. But we do not regard this as sufficient reason to scrap the use of a term if it is in fact most appropriate. The other objections to calling the product of SCNT an "embryo" are not about rhetoric and politics, but about the thing itself. They should be addressed.

First, "human embryo," in the traditional scientific definition of this term, refers to the earliest stages of human development, from the zygote through roughly eight weeks of gestation, after which time it is called a fetus. Because the product of SCNT is technically not a zygote, not having come from egg and sperm, it is argued that it cannot therefore be an embryo. Second, it is said that it cannot be an embryo because it is an "artifact," something produced entirely by human artifice, "made" rather than "begotten." Third, we do not yet know for sure whether this entity can in fact develop into a baby; hence, we do not *know* whether it has the full developmental potential of a human embryo formed by fertilization.

There are, however, good responses to these objections. The first product of SCNT is, on good biological grounds, quite properly regarded as the *equivalent* of a zygote, and its subsequent stages as *embryonic stages in development*. True, it is not technically "zygotic" in origin, and it owes its existence to human artifice. But these objections, dealing only with *origins*, ignore the organization and powers of this entity, and the crucially important fact of its capacity to undergo future embryological development—just like a sexually produced embryo. True, it originates as a result of human artifice, and it lacks the natural bi-parental (male-plus-female) precursors. But this particular "artifact" is alive and self-developing, and should it eventually give rise to a baby, that child would in its being and its capacities be indistinguishable from any other human being—hardly an artifact—in the same way that Dolly is a sheep. True, regarding its developmental potential, we do not yet have incontrovertible proof that a cloned human embryo can in fact do what embryos are "supposed" to do and what animal cloned embryos have already done, namely, develop into all the later stages of the organism, up to its full maturity (à la Dolly). But if we do not assume this last possibility—an assumption based on the biological continuity of all mammals*—there would be nothing to talk about in this whole matter of human cloning. As we emphasized in the first chapter of this report, *this entire inquiry assumes that cloned human embryos can someday be developed into live-born human beings.*

Once we make this assumption, neither its artificial nor its uniparental source alters the decisive point: the product of SCNT is an entity that is the first stage of a developing organism—of a determinate species (human), with a full genetic complement, and its own (albeit near-replicated) individual genetic identity. It hence deserves *on functional grounds* to be called an *embryo*. And that is the heart of the reason why we in this report shall call it an "embryo" (actually, for reasons soon to be discussed, a "*cloned* embryo"): because the decisive questions to be addressed in our moral reflections have to do not with the origin of the entity but with *its developmental potential*, its embryonic character must be kept centrally in mind.

This decision, based on what we believe comes closest to the truth about the product of SCNT, is supported by other, more practical considerations. We are disinclined to introduce other words to describe the early product of human cloning that might deprive discussion of the ethics of human cloning of its humanly significant context. Despite the novelty of cloning and its products, their con-

---

* A recent press report indicates that as-yet-unpublished work in China by Sheng Huizhen involved insertion of human somatic cell nuclei into enucleated rabbit eggs, and that the resulting cloned embryos developed to a stage where human embryonic stem cells could be isolated.[2] And, of course, in other mammals the product of SCNT has been grown all the way to live-born young that grow up to be able to produce young of their own.

siderable kinship to elements of normal reproduction and development means that we enter upon the discussion equipped with existing and relevant terms and notions. We do not start in a terminological vacuum or with an empty dictionary. We observe that even people who prefer not to call the one-celled product of SCNT a zygote or embryo use terms like "blastocyst" and "embryo" to name the product a few cell divisions later.* We think that using or coining other words will be more confusing to members of the public as they try to follow and contribute to the ethical discussion. And we clearly assume, as already stated, that the product of human SCNT could someday be shown to be capable of developing into a later-stage embryo, fetus, or live human being, even though such capacity has yet to be documented.

There are also very important *ethical* reasons that support our choice. We want to be very careful not to make matters easy for ourselves. We do not want to define away the moral questions of cloning-for-biomedical-research by denying to the morally crucial element a name that makes clear that there is a moral question to be faced. Yes, there is some ground for uncertainty about the being of the product of SCNT. Yet because something is ambiguous to *us* does not mean that it is ambiguous *in itself*. Where the moral stakes are high, we should not allow our uncertainty to lead us to

---

* Thus, for example, the report on *Scientific and Medical Aspects of Human Reproductive Cloning*, released by the National Academy of Sciences in January 2002, describes "nuclear transplantation to produce stem cells" as "a very different procedure" from what it calls "human reproductive cloning." Nevertheless, the report falls quite naturally into our normal way of speaking, a way that recognizes that the cloned product is, indeed, a human embryo and that any stem cells obtained from it would be *embryonic* stem cells. Thus, for example, the authors of the report can write a sentence such as the following (p. 2-6): "The experimental procedures required to produce stem cells through nuclear transplantation would consist of the transfer of a somatic cell nucleus from a patient into an enucleated egg, the in vitro culture of the embryo to the blastocyst stage, and the derivation of a pluripotent ES cell line from the inner cell mass of this blastocyst." Other scientists clearly insist that the primary product of SCNT is an embryo (see, for example, Dr. John Gearhart's presentation to the Council on embryonic stem cells, April 25, 2002; transcript on the Council's website, www.bioethics.gov).

regard the subject in question as being anything less than it might truly be.

The product of "SCNT" is not only an embryo; it is also a *clone*, genetically virtually identical to the individual that was the source of the transferred nucleus, hence an embryonic clone of the donor. There is, to be sure, much discussion about how close the genetic relation is between donor and embryonic clone, and about the phenotypic similarity of the clone to the donor.* Yet the goal in this process is in fact a blastocyst-stage cloned embryo (in the case of cloning-for-biomedical-research) or a child who is genetically virtually identical to the donor (in the case of cloning-to-produce-children); otherwise there would be no reason to produce a cloned embryo by SCNT rather than an (uncloned) embryo by ordinary IVF. A full and fitting name of the developing entity produced by human SCNT is "cloned human embryo," a term that also allows us to remember that, thanks to its peculiar origins, this embryo is not in all respects identical to an embryo produced by fertilization of egg by sperm.

As if things were not difficult enough, a further complication may soon arise, following reports of successful SCNT experiments in which human somatic cells were fused with *animal* oocytes, and the resulting product grown to the blastocyst stage of development. What are we to call the product of this kind of cloning? And what kind of species identity does it have? According to the advance reports (based on a presentation at a scientific meeting), the stem cells extracted from the blastocyst stage were demonstrated to be *human* stem cells (somewhat surprisingly, the mitochondria were also human in genotype). Is this, therefore, a cloned human em-

---

* The environment in which the donor came to be and lives surely differs from the one in which the cloned embryo may develop (if it does develop). There may be imprinting or epigenetic reprogramming differences in gene expression early on that may affect the physical and mental characteristics of the clone. There is also the matter of the mitochondrial genes (see Glossary of Terms), a small number of protein-producing genes out of a total of some 30,000 to 60,000, which are inherited from the female source of the egg (the clone would be genetically identical only in those cases in which the same woman donated both egg and somatic cell nucleus, to produce an embryonic clone of herself).

bryo? The only test that could settle the question—implantation into a woman's uterus for attempted gestation to see if a human child results—cannot ethically even be contemplated without already assuming a positive answer. In the face of uncertainty, therefore, and lest we err by overconfidence, there is *prima facie* reason to include even these cross-species entities in the category of "cloned human embryos." (When we come to the *ethical* issues of cloning-for-biomedical-research, we can consider whether this *terminological* judgment is matched by an *ethical* one.)

Conclusion

None of the terms available to us is entirely trouble-free. Yet the foregoing analysis leads us to the following conclusion regarding the terms best descriptive of the facts of the matter:

Human cloning (what it is): The asexual production of a new human organism that is, at all stages of development, genetically virtually identical to a currently existing or previously existing human being.

Human cloning (how it is done): It would be accomplished by introducing the nuclear material of a human somatic cell (donor) into an oocyte (egg) whose own nucleus has been removed or inactivated, yielding a product that has a human genetic constitution virtually identical to the donor of the somatic cell. This procedure is known as "somatic cell nuclear transfer" (SCNT).

Human cloning (why it is done): This same activity may be undertaken for purposes of producing children or for purposes of scientific and medical investigation and use, a distinction represented in the popular discussion by the terms "reproductive cloning" and "therapeutic cloning." We have chosen instead to use the following designations:

Cloning-to-produce-children: Production of a cloned human embryo, formed for the (proximate) purpose of initiating a pregnancy, with the (ultimate) goal of producing a child who will be genetically virtually identical to a currently existing or previously existing individual.

Cloning-for-biomedical-research: Production of a cloned human embryo, formed for the (proximate) purpose of using it in research or for extracting its stem cells, with the (ultimate) goals of gaining scientific knowledge of normal and abnormal development and of developing cures for human diseases.

Cloned human embryo: (a) The immediate and developing product of the initial act of cloning, accomplished by SCNT. (b) A human embryo resulting from the somatic cell nuclear transfer process (as contrasted with a human embryo arising from the union of egg and sperm).

ENDNOTES

[1] Vogelstein, B., et al., "Please don't call it cloning!" *Science*, 295: 1237, 2002.

[2] Leggett, K. and A. Regalado, "China Stem Cell Research Surges as Western Nations Ponder Ethics" *Wall Street Journal*, March 6, 2002, p. A1.

Chapter Four

Scientific Background

Introduction

The purpose of this chapter is to provide background on basic scientific aspects of human cloning for readers of this report. Background on stem cell research is also included to enable readers to understand how cloned embryos might be useful in stem cell and other biomedical research. This limited treatment only summarizes and highlights basic aspects of these topics, in part because two major detailed reports, *Scientific and Medical Aspects of Human Reproductive Cloning*[1] and *Stem Cells and the Future of Regenerative Medicine,*[2] have been recently published.

This review is based largely on scientific research papers published through June 2002, supplemented by references to several articles in the popular press. However, the research areas of cloning and stem cell research are being very actively investigated, and significant new developments are published frequently. Publication of new results could change some of the interpretations and emphases in this review.

Use of unfamiliar technical terms has been avoided wherever possible. Scientific names and terms used are described and defined in the Glossary of Terms.

Some Basic Facts about Human Cell Biology and Sexual Reproduction

We begin with some basic facts about human cells, germ cells (egg and sperm), and early embryonic development to provide the background for understanding the mechanism of cloning and the differences between sexual and asexual reproduction.

Normal human cells with nuclei contain forty-six chromosomes, twenty-two pairs plus two X chromosomes if the individual is female, or twenty-two pairs plus one X and one Y chromosome if the individual is male. These chromosomes contain nearly all of the cell's DNA and, therefore, the genes of the cell. During formation of sperm cells, a process of specialized cell division produces mature sperm cells containing twenty-three chromosomes (twenty-two unpaired chromosomes plus either X or Y). During the formation of eggs (oocytes), a process of specialized cell division produces a cell containing two pronuclei, each of which contains twenty-two unpaired chromosomes plus an X. During fertilization, a polar body containing one of these pronuclei is ejected from the egg.

Fusion of egg and sperm cells and the subsequent fusion of their nuclei (the defining acts of all sexual reproduction) produce a zygote that again contains a nucleus with the adult cell complement of forty-six chromosomes, half from each parent [See Figure 1]. The zygote then begins the gradual process of cell division, growth, and differentiation. After four to five days, the developing embryo attains the 100-200 cell (blastocyst) stage. In normal reproduction, the blastocyst implants into the wall of the uterus, where, suitably nourished, it continues the process of coordinated cell, tissue, and organ differentiation that eventually produces the organized, articulated, and integrated whole that is the newborn infant. According to some estimates, about half of all early human embryos fail to implant, and are expelled with the menses during the next menstrual cycle.

Not quite all the DNA of a human cell resides in its nucleus. All human cells, including eggs and sperm, contain small, energy-producing organelles called mitochondria. Mitochondria contain a small piece of DNA that specifies the genetic instructions for making several essential mitochondrial proteins. When additional mitochondria are produced in the cell, the mitochondrial DNA is replicated, and a copy of it is passed along to the new mitochondria that are formed. During fertilization, sperm mitochondria are selectively degraded inside the zygote. Thus, the developing embryo inherits solely or principally mitochondria (and mitochondrial DNA) from the egg.

Human reproduction has also been accomplished with the help of in vitro fertilization (IVF) of eggs by sperm, and the subsequent transfer of one or more early embryos to a woman for gestation and birth. Even though such union of egg and sperm requires laboratory assistance and takes place outside of the body, human reproduction using IVF is still sexual in the biological sense: the new human being arises from two biological parents through the union of egg and sperm.

Egg and sperm cells combined in vitro have also been used to start the process of animal development. Transfer of the resulting blastocysts into the uterus of a female of the appropriate animal species is widely used in animal husbandry with resulting successful live births.

Cloning (Asexual Reproduction) of Mammals

The startling announcement that Dolly the sheep had been produced by cloning[3] indicated that it was possible to produce live mammalian offspring via asexual reproduction through cloning with adult donor cell nuclei.[*] In outline form, the steps used to produce live offspring in the mammalian species that have been cloned so far are:

---

[*] Previous experiments dating from the 1950s had shown that it was possible to clone amphibians. Earlier experiments had also produced clones of animals using *embryonic* donor cells. What made the report of Dolly's birth stand out was the fact that a mammal had been cloned, and from cells taken from an adult.

1. Obtain an egg cell from a female of a mammalian species.

2. Remove the nuclear DNA from the egg cell, to produce an enucleated egg.

3. Insert the nucleus of a donor adult cell into the enucleated egg, to produce a reconstructed egg.

4. Activate the reconstructed egg with chemicals or electric current, to stimulate the reconstructed egg to commence cell division.

5. Sustain development of the cloned embryo to a suitable stage in vitro, and then transfer the resulting cloned embryo to the uterus of a female host that has been suitably prepared to receive it.

6. Bring to live birth a cloned animal that is genetically virtually identical (except for the mitochondrial DNA) to the animal that donated the adult cell nucleus.

Cloning to produce live offspring carries with it several possibilities not available through sexual reproduction. Because the number of presumably identical donor cells is very large, this process could produce a very large number of genetically virtually identical individuals, limited only by the supply of eggs and female animals that could bear the young. In principle, any animal, male or female, newborn or adult, could be cloned, and in any quantity. Because mammalian cells can be frozen and stored for prolonged periods at low temperature and grown again for use as donor cells in cloning, one may even clone individuals who have died. In theory, a clone could be cloned again, on and on, without limit. In mice, such "cloning of clones" has extended out to six generations.[4]

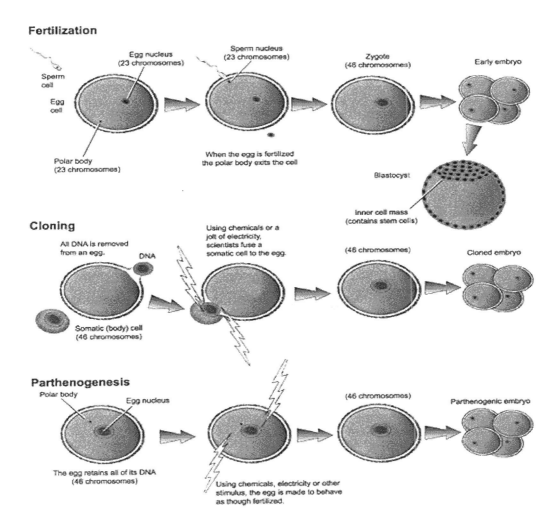

Figure 1: Diagram of early stages of human fertilization, cloning, and parthenogenesis.

[Modified from Rick Weiss and Patterson Clark, *The Washington Post.*]

Since the report of the birth of Dolly the cloned sheep, attempts have been made to clone at least nine other mammalian species. As summarized in Table 1, live offspring have been produced in a low percentage of cloned embryo transfer experiments with sheep, cattle, goats, mice, pigs, cats[5] and rabbits.[6] According to a press report,[7] attempts to clone rats, dogs, and primates using adult cell DNA have not yet yielded live offspring. In experiments to clone different mammalian species, many of the transferred cloned embryos fail to develop normally and abort spontaneously in utero. In addition, a variety of health problems have been reported in many of the cloned animals that survived to live birth.[8] However, some surviving cloned cattle appear physiologically similar to their uncloned counterparts, and two cloned cows have given birth to their own offspring.[9,10]

Why is production of live cloned mammalian offspring a relatively rare event? Several factors may play a role. Enucleation of the egg may (variably from one attempt to the next) remove or damage its "epigenetic reprogramming" (see Glossary of Terms) capabilities. Isolating a nucleus from the donor cell and manipulating it to insert it into the egg is also a traumatic process that may damage the nucleus. An optimal in vitro nutritive environment for the development of cloned animal embryos may not yet have been determined. One interpretation[11] attributes the early death of many cloned embryos to complete failure or incompleteness of epigenetic reprogramming.

Epigenetic Modification and Reprogramming

Normal mammalian embryonic development results from selective expression of some genes and repression of others. Tissue differentiation depends upon several types of "epigenetic modifications" (see Glossary of Terms) of DNA structure and spatial organization that selectively turn genes on and off. The chromosomal DNAs of egg and sperm cells are modified during their

TABLE 1. SOME COMPARATIVE DATA ON LIVE BIRTHS FROM CLONING OF ANIMALS

[For a more complete collection of data, see the NAS Report *Scientific and Medical Aspects of Human Cloning*]

Animal Species	Donor Cell	Number of Cloned Embryos Transferred	Number of Live Births	Live Births per Embryo Transfer	Reference
Sheep	udder cells (frozen)	29	1	3.4%	1
Cattle	fetal fibroblasts	496	24-30#	4.8-6%	2a
	cumulus & oviduct cells	10	4-8*	40-80%	2b
Mice	cumulus cells	2468	31**	1.3%	3
Goats	transgenic fetal fibroblasts	97	5	5.2%	4a
	fetal fibroblasts	85	3	3.5%	4b
	transgenic fetal fibroblasts	184	5	2.7%	4c
Pigs	fetal fibroblasts	110	1	0.9%	5a
		335	5	1.5%	5b
Cats	cumulus cells	87	1	1.1%	6
Rabbits	cumulus cells	371	6	1.6%	7

References:
1. Wilmut, I., et al., Nature, 385: 264-267 (1997)
2a. Cibelli, J.B., et al., Science, 280: 1256-1258 (1998)
2b. Kato, Y., et al., Science, 282: 2095-2098 (1998)
3. Wakayama, T., et al., Nature, 394: 369-374 (1998)
4a. Baguisi, A., et al., Nature Biotechnology, 17: 456-461 (1999)
4b. Keefer, C.L., et al., Biol Reprod, 64: 849-856 (2001)
4c. Reggio, B.C., et al., Biol Reprod, 65: 1528-33 (2001)
5a. Onishi, A., et al., Science, 289: 1188-90 (2000)
5b. Polejaeva, I.A., et al., Nature, 407: 86-90 (2000)
6. Shin, T., et al., Nature, 415: 859 (2002)
7. Chesne, P., et al., Nature Biotechnology, 20: 366-369 (2002)

Six animals died shortly after birth; * four animals died shortly after birth;
** 20 animals died at a young age [Ogonuki, N.K., et al., Nature Genetics, 30: 253-4 (2002)].

maturation, so that at fertilization, both sets of DNA are ready for the complex pattern of gene expression required for normal embryonic development. In order for the DNA of a differentiated *adult* cell to direct embryonic development in cloning, it must be "epigenetically reprogrammed." That is, the epigenetic modifications that allowed the cell to express genes appropriate for, for example, a differentiated skin cell must be reduced, and the gene expression program required for full embryonic development must be activated.

During cloning, cytoplasmic factors in the egg cell reprogram the chromosomal DNA of the somatic cell. In rare cases, this reprogramming is sufficient to enable embryonic development to proceed all the way to the birth of a live animal (for examples, see Table 1). In many cloning experiments, epigenetic reprogramming probably fails or is abnormal, and the developing animal dies. Incomplete epigenetic reprogramming could also explain why some live-born cloned animals suffer from subtle defects that sometimes do not appear for years.[12]

The completeness of epigenetic reprogramming is crucial for successful cloning-to-produce-children. It will also be important to assess the impact of variation in epigenetic reprogramming on the biological properties of cloned stem cell preparations. If the extent of epigenetic reprogramming varies from one cloning event to the next, the protein expression pattern and thus the biological properties of cloned stem cell preparations may also vary. Thus, it may be necessary to produce and test multiple cloned stem cell preparations before preparations that are informative about human disease or useful in cellular transplantation therapies can be identified.

Cloning-to-Produce-Children

At this writing, it is uncertain whether anyone has attempted cloning-to-produce-children. Although claims of such attempts have been reported in the press,[13,14] no credible evidence of any such experiments has been reported as of June 2002. Thus, it is not yet known whether a transferred cloned human embryo can progress all the way to live birth. However, the steps in such an experiment would probably be similar to those described for animal cloning [see above and references to Table 1]. After a thorough review of the data on animal cloning, the NAS panel, in its report *Scientific and Medical Aspects of Human Cloning* [page ES-1], came to the following conclusion: "It [cloning-to-produce-children] is dangerous and likely to fail."

Stem Cells and Regenerative Medicine

The subject of stem cell research is much too large to be covered extensively here. Yet the following information on stem cells and their possible uses in medical treatments should facilitate understanding of the relationships between cloning-for-biomedical-research and stem cells (see also the reports *Scientific and Medical Aspects of Human Reproductive Cloning* and *Stem Cells and the Future of Regenerative Medicine*).

Stem cells are undifferentiated multipotent precursor cells that are capable both of perpetuating themselves as stem cells and of undergoing differentiation into one or more specialized types of cells (for example, kidney, muscle). Human embryonic stem cells have been isolated from embryos at the blastocyst stage[15] or from the germinal tissue of fetuses.[16] Multipotent adult progenitor cells have been isolated from sources such as human[17] and rodent[18] bone marrow. Such cell populations can be differentiated in vitro into a number of different cell types, and thus are the subject of much current research into their possible uses in regenerative medicine. Cloned human embryonic stem cell preparations could be produced using somatic cell nuclear transfer to produce a cloned human embryo, and then taking it apart at the (100-200 cell) blastocyst stage and isolating stem cells (see Figure 2). These stem cells would be genetically virtually identical to cells from the nucleus donor.

Scientists are pursuing the development of therapies based on transplantation of cells for several human diseases, including Parkinson's disease and Type I diabetes. In Parkinson's disease, particular brain cells that produce the essential neurotransmitter dopamine die selectively. Experimental clinical treatment involving transplantation of human *fetal* brain cell populations, in which a small fraction of the cells produce dopamine, has improved the condition of some Parkinson's disease patients.[19] Dopamine-producing neurons derived from mouse embryonic stem cells have been shown to function in an animal model of Parkinson's disease.[20] Thus, there is a possibility that transplantation of dopamine-producing neural cells derived from embryonic or adult stem cell populations might be a useful treatment for Parkinson's disease in the future.

However, to be effective as long-term treatments of Parkinson's disease, Type I diabetes, and other diseases, cell transplantation therapies will have to overcome the immune rejection problem. Cells from one person transplanted into the body of another are usually recognized as foreign and killed by the immune system. If cells derived from stem cell preparations are to be broadly useful in transplantation therapies for human diseases, some way or ways around this problem will have to be found. For example, if the cells were isolated from a cloned human embryo at the blastocyst stage, in which the donor nucleus came from a patient with Parkinson's disease, in theory these stem cells would produce the same proteins as the patient. The hope is that dopamine-producing cells derived from these "individualized" stem cell preparations would not be immunologically rejected upon transplantation back into the Parkinson's disease patient. Alternatively, if dopamine-producing cells could be derived from the patient's own adult stem cell or multipotent adult precursor cell populations, they could also be used in such therapies. Another possibility is mentioned in a press report[21] about work with a single Parkinson's disease patient, in which brain cells were removed from the patient, expanded by growth in vitro, stimulated to increase dopamine production, and transplanted back into the brain of the same patient with an observed reduction in disease symptoms.

By combining specific gene modification and cloned stem cell procedures, Rideout et al.[22] have provided a remarkable example of how some human genetic diseases might someday be treated.

Starting with a mouse strain that was deficient in immune system function because of a gene mutation, these investigators (1) produced a cloned stem cell line carrying the gene mutation, (2) specifically repaired the gene mutation in vitro, (3) differentiated the repaired cloned stem cell preparation in vitro into bone marrow precursor cells, and (4) treated the mutant mice with the repaired bone marrow precursor cells and observed a restoration of immune cell function.

Although remarkably successful, the experimental results included a caveat. The investigators also observed a tendency of even these cloned bone marrow precursor cells to be recognized as foreign by the recipient mice. Rideout et al. were led to conclude: "Our results raise the provocative possibility that even genetically matched cells derived by therapeutic cloning may still face barriers to effective transplantation for some disorders."

Lanza et al.[23] have also evaluated the potential for immune rejection of cloned embryonic materials, while showing the potential therapeutic value of tissues taken from cloned fetuses. Cloned cattle embryos at the blastocyst stage were transferred to the uteri of surrogate mothers and allowed to develop for five to eight weeks. Fetal heart, kidney, and skeletal muscle tissues were isolated, and degradable polymer vehicles containing these cloned cells were then transplanted back into the animals that donated the nuclei for cloning. The investigators observed no rejection reaction to the transplanted cloned cells using two different immunological tests. More investigations with cloned stem cell materials involving different stem cell preparations of varying sizes, different sites of implantation, and sensitive tests to detect low levels of immunological rejection will be required for a complete assessment of the possibility of using cloned stem cell populations to solve the immune rejection problem.

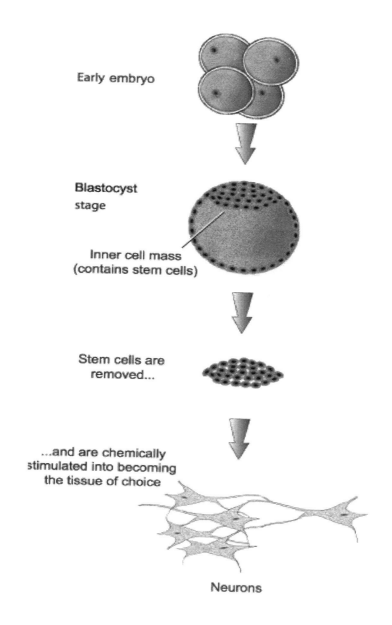

Figure 2: Stages in the development, isolation, and transformation of embryonic stem cells.

[Modified from Rick Weiss and Patterson Clark, *The Washington Post.*]

Human Cloning-for-Biomedical-Research

Producing cloned stem cell preparations for possible use in individual patients suffering from diseases like Parkinson's disease and Type I diabetes is one reason to pursue cloning-for-biomedical-research.[24] In vitro production of cloned human embryos could also be important to scientists interested in studying early human development. Stem cells derived from cloned human embryos at the blastocyst stage that were produced with nuclei from individuals with genetic diseases could be useful in the study of the critical events that lead to these diseases (for example, see Bahn et al.[25]). Specific genes could be introduced into developing human embryos to obtain information about the role or roles of these genes in early human development.

One attempt at human cloning-for-biomedical-research has been published in the scientific literature by Cibelli et al.[26] as of the end of June 2002.* It involved the following steps (see Figure 1):

1. Obtain human eggs from informed and consenting female volunteers.

2. Remove the nuclear DNA from the egg cell, to produce an enucleated egg.

3. Insert the nucleus of a cell from an informed and consenting adult donor into the enucleated egg, to produce a reconstituted egg.

---

* According to a press report (Hall, C.T., "UCSF Admits Human Clone Research: Work to Duplicate Embryos for Medical Purposes on Hold" *San Francisco Chronicle*, May 25, 2002, p. A1), other attempts to produce cloned human embryos for biomedical research were carried out at the University of California-San Francisco by Roger Pedersen and coworkers in 1999 and 2001. Another press report (Leggett K., and A., Regalado "China Stem Cell Research Surges as Western Nations Ponder Ethics," *Wall Street Journal*, March 6, 2002, p. A1) indicates that as-yet-unpublished work in China by Sheng Huizhen involved insertion of human somatic cell nuclei into enucleated rabbit eggs, and that the resulting cloned embryos developed to a stage where human embryonic stem cells could be isolated.

4. Activate the reconstituted egg with chemicals or electricity to stimulate it to commence cell division in vitro, producing a cloned embryo.

5. Use a microscope to follow the early cell divisions of the cloned embryo.

In the experiments described by Cibelli et al., the stated intent was to create cloned human embryos that would progress to the 100-200 cell stage, at which point the cloned embryo would be taken apart, stem cells would be isolated from the inner cell mass, and an attempt would be made to grow and preserve "individualized" human stem cells (see Figure 2) for the possible future medical benefit of the somatic cell donor. Because the cloned human embryos stopped dividing and died at the six-cell stage, no stem cells were isolated in these experiments. In light of results in other animal species and the variable completeness of "epigenetic reprogramming," it is perhaps not surprising that sixteen of the nineteen cloned human embryos described by Cibelli et. al. did not undergo cell division and none of the other three divided beyond the six-cell stage.

Although the steps these researchers followed in these experiments were the same as those that would be used by those attempting human cloning-to-produce-children, they distinguished their intent from such cloning by stating: "Strict guidelines for the conduct of this research have been established by Advanced Cell Technology's independent Ethics Advisory Board (EAB). In order to prevent any possibility of reproductive cloning, the EAB requires careful accounting of all eggs and embryos used in the research. No embryo created by means of NT [nuclear transfer] technology may be maintained beyond 14 days of development."

Parthenogenesis (Another Form of Asexual Reproduction)

Using chemical or electrical stimuli, it is also possible to stimulate human eggs to undergo several rounds of cell division, as if they had been fertilized (see Figure 1). In this case, the egg retains all forty-six egg cell chromosomes and egg cell mitochondria. In amphibians, this asexual reproduction process, known as parthenogenesis, has produced live offspring that contain the same nuclear DNA as the egg. These offspring are all necessarily female. Parthenogenesis in mammals has not led reproducibly to the production of live offspring.[27]

Cibelli et al.[26] activated human eggs (obtained from informed and consenting donors) by parthenogenesis, and obtained multiple cell divisions up to the early embryo stage in six out of twenty-two attempts. Although there was no report that stem cells were isolated in these experiments, it is possible that parthenogenesis of human eggs could induce them to develop to a stage where parthenogenetic stem cells could be isolated. For example, Cibelli et al.[28] derived a monkey parthenogenetic stem cell preparation from *Macaca fasicularis* eggs activated by parthenogenesis. Whether cloned stem cells resulting from parthenogenesis have been completely and correctly epigenetically reprogrammed remains to be determined.

ENDNOTES

1 National Academy of Sciences (NAS). *Scientific and Medical Aspects of Human Reproductive Cloning,* Washington, DC. National Academy Press, 2002.

2 National Research Council/Institute of Medicine (NRC/IOM). *Stem Cells and the Future of Regenerative Medicine.* Washington DC. National Academy Press, 2001.

3 Wilmut, I., et al. "Viable offspring derived from fetal and adult mammalian cells" *Nature,* 385: 810-813, 1997.

4 Wakayama, T., et al. "Cloning of mice to six generations" *Nature,* 407: 318-319, 2000.

5 Shin, T., et al. "A cat cloned by nuclear transplantation" *Nature,* 415: 859, 2002.

6 Chesne, P., et al. "Cloned rabbits produced by nuclear transfer from adult somatic cells" *Nature Biotechnology*, 20: 366-369, 2002.

7 Kolata, G. "In Cloning, Failure Far Exceeds Success" *New York Times*, December 11, 2001, page D1.

8 See Table 2 in Reference 1.

9 Lanza, R.P., et al. "Cloned cattle can be healthy and normal," *Science*, 294: 1893-1894, 2001.

10 Cibelli, J.B., et al. "The health profile of cloned animals" *Nature Biotechnology*, 20: 13-14, 2002.

11 Rideout III, W.M., et al. "Nuclear cloning and epigenetic reprogramming of the genome" *Science*, 293: 1093-1098, 2001.

12 Ogonuki, N., et al. "Early death of mice cloned from somatic cells" *Nature Genetics*, 30: 253-254, 2002.

13 Weiss, R. "Human Cloning Bid Stirs Experts' Anger; Problems in Animal Cases Noted" *The Washington Post*, April 11, 2001, page A1.

14 Brown, D. "Human Clone's Birth Predicted; Delivery Outside U.S. May Come By 2003, Researcher Says" *The Washington Post*, May 16, 2002, p. A8.

15 Thomson, J.A., et al. "Embryonic stem cell lines derived from human blastocysts" *Science*, 282: 1145-1147, 1998.

16 Shamblott, M.J., et al. "Derivation of pluripotent stem cells from cultured human primordial germ cells" *Proc Nat Acad Sci U.S.A.*, 95: 13726-13731, 1998.

17 Reyes, M., et al. "Origin of endothelial progenitors in human postnatal bone marrow" *Journal of Clinical Investigation*, 109: 337-346, 2002.

18 Jiang, Y., et al. "Pluripotency of mesenchymal stem cells derived from adult marrow," *Nature*, 418: 41-49, 2002.

19 Hagell, P., and P. Brundin, "Cell survival and clinical outcome following intrastriatal transplantation in Parkinson's disease" *J Neuropathol Exp Neurol*, 60: 741-752, 2001.

20 Kim, J-H., et al. "Dopamine neurons derived from embryonic stem cells function in an animal model of Parkinson's disease" *Nature* 418: 50-56, 2002.

21 Weiss, R. "Stem Cell Transplant Works in Calif. Case, Parkinson's Traits Largely Disappear," *The Washington Post,* April 9, 2002, p. A8.

22 Rideout III, W.M., et al. "Correction of a genetic defect by nuclear transplantation and combined cell and gene therapy" *Cell,* 109: 17-27, 2002.

23 Lanza, R.P., et al. "Generation of histocompatible tissues using nuclear transplantation" *Nature Biotechnology,* 20: 689-696, 2002.

24 Lanza, R.P., et al. "Human therapeutic cloning" *Nature Medicine,* 5: 975-977, 1999.

25 Bahn, S., et al. "Neuronal target genes of the neuron-restrictive silencer factor in neurospheres derived from fetuses with Down's syndrome: A gene expression study" *The Lancet,* 359: 310-315, 2002.

26 Cibelli, J.B., et al. "Somatic cell nuclear transfer in humans: Pronuclear and early embryonic development" e-biomed: *The Journal of Regenerative Medicine,* 2: 25-31, 2001.

27 Rougier, N., and Z. Werb. "Minireview: Parthenogenesis in mammals" *Mol Reprod Devel* 59: 468-474, 2001.

28 Cibelli, J.B., et al. "Parthenogenetic stem cells in nonhuman primates" *Science,* 295: 819, 2002.

Chapter Five

The Ethics of Cloning-to-Produce-Children

Cloning-to-produce-children has been the subject of two major national reports in recent years—first by the National Bioethics Advisory Commission in June 1997,[1] and more recently by the National Academy of Sciences in January 2002.[2] Both reports concluded that attempts to clone a human being "at this time" would be unethical, owing to questions about the safety of the technique and the likelihood of physical harm to those involved. But both reports also concluded that the nation required much deeper reflection about the "ethical and social implications" of cloning-to-produce-children beyond the scientific and medical aspects of the procedure. As the National Academy of Sciences report stated:

> Our present opposition to human reproductive cloning is based on science and medicine, irrespective of broader considerations. The panel stresses, however, that a broad ethical debate must be encouraged so that the public can be prepared to make decisions if human reproductive cloning is some day considered medically safe for mothers and offspring.[3]

In this chapter we attempt to take up this charge to engage in a broad ethical consideration of the merits of cloning-to-produce-children.

The prospect of cloning-to-produce-children raises a host of moral questions, among them the following: Could the first attempts to clone a human child be made without violating accepted moral norms governing experimentation on human subjects? What harms might be inflicted on the cloned child as a consequence of having been made a clone? Is it significant that the cloned child would inherit a genetic identity lived in advance by another—and, in some cases, the genetic identity of the cloned child's rearing parent? Is it significant that cloned children would be the first human beings whose genetic identity was entirely known and selected in advance? How might cloning-to-produce-children affect relationships within the cloning families? More generally, how might it affect the relationship between the generations? How might it affect the way society comes to view children? What other prospects would we be tacitly approving in advance by accepting this practice? What important human goods might be enhanced or sacrificed were we to approve cloning-to-produce-children?

In what follows, we shall explicitly consider many of these questions. But as we do so, we shall not lose sight of the larger and fundamental human contexts discussed in Chapter One—namely, the meaning of human procreation and care of children, the means and ends of biotechnology, and the relation between science and society. Indeed, overarching our entire discussion of the *specific* ethical issues is our concern for the human significance of procreation as a whole and our desire to protect what is valuable in it from erosion and degradation—not just from cloning but from other possible technological and nontechnological dangers. Readers of this report are encouraged to consider the discussion that follows in a similar light.

We will begin by formulating the best moral case for cloning-to-produce-children—describing both the specific purposes it might serve and the philosophic and moral arguments made in its favor. From there we will move to the moral case against cloning-to-produce-children. Beginning with the safety objections that have dominated the debate thus far, we will show how these concerns ultimately point beyond themselves toward broader ethical concerns. Chief among these is how cloning-to-produce-children would challenge the basic nature of human procreation and the meaning of having children. We shall also consider cloning's effects on human identity, how it might move procreation toward a form of manufacture or toward eugenics, and how it could distort family relations and affect society as a whole.

*   *   *

I. The Case for Cloning-to-Produce-Children

Arguments in defense of cloning-to-produce-children often address questions of reproduction, but they tend to focus on only a relatively narrow sliver of the goods and principles involved. This certainly does not mean that such arguments lack merit. Indeed, some of the arguments in favor of cloning-to-produce-children appeal to the deepest and most meaningful of our society's shared values.

A. Purposes

In recent years, in anticipation of cloning-to-produce-children, proponents have articulated a variety of possible uses of a perfected technology: providing a "biologically related child" for an infertile couple; permitting reproduction for single individuals or same-sex couples; avoiding the risk of genetic disease; securing a genetically identical source of organs or tissues perfectly suitable for transplantation; "replacing" a loved spouse or child who is dying or has died; obtaining a child with a genotype of one's own choosing (including one's own genotype); replicating individuals of great genius, talent, or beauty, or individuals possessing traits that are for other reasons attractive to the cloners; and creating sets of genetically identical humans who might have special advantages in highly cooperative ventures in both war and peace.[4] The desire to control or select the genomes of children-to-be through cloning has charmed more than a few prospective users, in the United States and around the world.

Although we appreciate that a perfected technology, once introduced for one purpose, might then be used for any of these purposes, we shall examine further only those stated purposes that seem to us to merit serious consideration.

1. To Produce Biologically Related Children

Human cloning would allow individuals or couples with fertility problems to have biologically related children. For example, if a man could not produce sperm, cloning would allow him to have a child who is "biologically related" to him. In addition, it would allow married couples with fertility problems to avoid using donor gametes, and therefore avoid raising children with genetic inheritances from outside the marriage.

2. To Avoid Genetic Disease

Human cloning could allow couples at risk of generating children with genetic disease to have healthy children. For example, if both parents carried one copy of a recessive gene for the same heritable disorder, cloning might allow them to ensure that their child does not inherit the known genetic disease (without having to resort to using donor gametes or practicing preimplantation or prenatal genetic diagnosis and elimination of afflicted embryos or fetuses).

3. To Obtain "Rejection-Proof" Transplants

Human cloning could produce ideal transplant donors for people who are sick or dying. For example, if no genetic match could be found for a sick child needing a kidney or bone marrow transplant, and the parents had planned to have another child, cloning could potentially serve the human goods of beginning a new life and saving an existing one.

4. To "Replicate" a Loved One

Human cloning would allow parents to "replicate" a dead or dying child or relative. For example, one can imagine a case in which a family—mother, father, and child—is involved in a terrible car accident in which the father dies instantly and the child is critically injured. The mother, told that her child will soon die, decides that the best way to redeem the tragedy is to clone her dying child. This would allow her to preserve a connection with both her dead husband and her dying child, to create new life as a partial human answer to the grievous misfortune of her child's untimely death, and to continue the name and biological lineage of her deceased husband.

5. To Reproduce Individuals of Great Genius, Talent, or Beauty

Human cloning would allow families or society to reproduce individuals of great genius, talent, or beauty, where these traits are presumed to be based on the individuals' desirable or superior genetic makeups. For example, some admirers of great athletes, musicians, or mathematicians, believing that the admired attributes are the result of a superior genetic endowment, might want to clone these distinguished individuals. Just as the cloning of cattle is being promoted as a means of perpetuating champion milk- or meat-producing cows, so cloning-to-produce-children has been touted as a means of perpetuating certain "superior" human exemplars.

B. Arguments

The purposes or reasons for cloning-to-produce-children are, as they are stated, clearly intelligible on their face. When challenged, the defenders of these purposes often appeal to larger moral and political goods. These typically fall within the following three categories: human freedom, existence, and well-being.

1. The Goodness of Human Freedom

Strictly speaking, the appeal to human freedom is not so much a defense of cloning itself as it is of the *right* to practice it, asserted against those who seek to prohibit it. No one, we suspect, would say that he wanted to clone himself or any one else in order to be free or to vindicate the goodness of liberty. Nevertheless, human freedom is a defense often heard in support of a "right" to clone.

Those who defend cloning-to-produce-children on the grounds of human freedom make two kinds of arguments. The first is that because individuals in pluralistic societies have different definitions of the good life and of right and wrong, society must protect individual freedom to choose against the possible tyranny of the majority. This means securing and even expanding the rights of individuals to make choices so long as their choices do not directly infringe on the rights (and especially the physical safety) of other rights-bearing citizens. In *Eisenstadt v. Baird* (1972), the United States Supreme Court enunciated what has been called a principle of reproductive freedom: "If the right to privacy means anything, it is the right of the individual, married or single, to be free from unwarranted governmental intrusion into matters so affecting a person as a decision whether to bear or beget a child."[5] Defenders of cloning-to-produce-children argue that, in the event that the physical risks to mother and future child were shown to be ethically acceptable, the use of this new reproductive technology would fall under the protective umbrella of reproductive freedom.

A second defense of human cloning on the grounds of freedom is the claim that human existence is by its very nature "open-ended," "indeterminate," and "unpredictable." Human beings are always remaking themselves, their values, and their ways of interacting with one another. New technologies are central to this open-ended idea of human life, and to shut down such technologies simply because they change the "traditional" ways of doing things is unjustifiable. As constitutional scholar Laurence Tribe has argued in reference to human cloning: "A society that bans acts of human creation that reflect unconventional sex roles or parenting models (surrogate motherhood, in vitro fertilization, artificial insemination, and the like) for no better reason than that such acts dare to defy 'nature' and tradition (and to risk adding to life's complexity) is a society that risks cutting itself off from vital experimentation and risks sterilizing a significant part of its capacity to grow."[6]

2. The Goodness of Existence

Like the appeal to freedom, the appeal to the goodness of existence is not an argument *for* cloning, but an argument *against* opponents who speak up in the name of protecting the cloned child-to-be against the harms connected with its risky and strange origins as a clone. This argument asserts that attempts to produce children through cloning, like *any* attempt to produce a child, will directly benefit the cloned-child-to-be, since without the act of cloning the child in question would not exist. Existence itself, it is argued, is the first "interest" that makes all other interests—including the interests of safety and well-being—possible. Even taking into account the possibility of serious genetic or developmental disorders, this position holds that a cloned individual, once born, would prefer existence as a clone to no existence at all. There is also a serious corollary about how, in the absence of a principle that values existence *as such*, we will and should regard and treat people born with disabilities or deformities: opponents of cloning might appear in a position of intolerance—of saying to cloned individuals, "Better for us (and for you) had you never existed."

3. The Goodness of Well-Being

The third moral argument for cloning-to-produce-children is that it would contribute in certain cases to the fulfillment of human goods that are widely honored and deeply rooted in modern democratic society. These human goods include the health of newborn and existing children, reproductive possibilities for infertile couples, and the possibility of having a biologically related child. In all these circumstances, human cloning could relieve existing suffering and sorrow or prevent them in the future. Those who take this position do not necessarily defend human cloning-to-produce-children as such. Rather, they argue that a moral and practical line can be drawn between cloning-to-produce-children that serves the "therapeutic" aims of health (for the cloned child-to-be, for the infertile couple, or for an existing child) and the "eugenic" aims of producing or mass-producing superior people.

Some people argue more broadly that an existing generation has a responsibility to ensure, to the extent possible, the genetic quality and fitness of the next generation. Human cloning, they argue, offers a new method for human control and self-improvement, by allowing families to have children free of specific genetic diseases or society to reproduce children with superior genetic endowments. It also provides a new means for gaining knowledge about the age-old question of nature versus nurture in contributing to human achievement and human flourishing, and to see how clones of great geniuses measure up against the "originals."

C. Critique and Conclusion

While we as a Council acknowledge merit in some of the arguments made for cloning-to-produce-children, we are generally not persuaded by them. The fundamental weakness of the proponents' case is found in their incomplete view of human procreation and families, and especially the place and well-being of children. Proponents of cloning tend to see procreation primarily as the free exercise of a parental right, namely, a right to satisfy parental desires for self-fulfillment or a right to have a child who is healthy or "superior." Parents seek to overcome obstacles to reproduction, to keep their children free of genetic disease or disorder, and to provide them with the best possible genetic endowment. The principles guiding such prospective parents are freedom (for themselves), control (over their child), and well-being (both for themselves and what they imagine is best for their child). Even taken together, these principles provide at best only a partial understanding of the meaning and entailments of human procreation and child-rearing. In practice, they may prove to undermine the very goods that the proponents of cloning aim to serve, by undermining the unconditional acceptance of one's offspring that is so central to parenthood.

There are a number of objections—or at the very least limitations—to viewing cloning-to-produce-children through the prism of rights. Basic human rights are usually asserted on behalf of the human individual agent: for example, a meaningful right *not to be prevented* from bearing a child can be asserted for each individual against state-mandated sterilization programs. But the act of procreation is not an act involving a single individual. Indeed, until human cloning arrives, it continues to be impossible for any one person to procreate alone. More important, there is a crucial third party involved: the child, whose centrality to the activity exposes the insufficiency of thinking about procreation in terms of rights.

After all, rights are limited in the following crucial way: they cannot be ethically exercised at the expense of the rights of another. But the "right to reproduce" cannot be ethically exercised without at least considering the child that such exercise will bring into being and who is at risk of harm and injustice from the exercise. This obligation cannot be waived by an appeal to the absolutist argument of the goodness of existence. Yes, existence is a primary good, but that does not diminish the ethical significance of knowingly and willfully putting a child in grave physical danger in the very act of giving that child existence. It is certainly true that a life with even severe disability may well be judged worth living by its bearer: "It is better to have been born as I am than not to be here at all." But if his or her disability was caused by behavior that could have been avoided by parents (for example, by not drinking or using drugs during pregnancy, or, arguably, by not cloning), many would argue that they should have avoided it. A post-facto affirmation of existence by the harmed child would not retroactively excuse the parental misconduct that caused the child's disability, nor would it justify their failure to think of the child's well-being as they went about exercising their "right to procreate." Indeed, procreation is, by its very nature, a limitation of absolute rights, since it brings into existence another human being toward whom we have responsibilities and duties.

In short, the right to decide *"whether* to bear or beget a child" does not include a right to have a child *by whatever means*. Nor can this right be said to imply a corollary—the right to decide what *kind* of child one is going to have. There are at least some circumstances where reproductive freedom must be limited to protect the good of the child (as, for instance, with the ban on incest). Our society's commitment to freedom and parental authority by no means implies that all innovative procedures and practices should be allowed or accepted, no matter how bizarre or dangerous.

Proponents of cloning, when they do take into account the interests of the child, sometimes argue that this interest justifies and even requires thoroughgoing parental control over the procreative process. Yet this approach, even when well-intentioned, may undermine the good of the child more than it serves the child's best interests. For one thing, cloning-to-produce-children of a desired or worthy sort overlooks the need to restrain the parental temptation to total mastery over children. It is especially morally dubious for this project to go forward when we know so little about the unforeseen and unintended consequences of exercising such genetic control. In trying by cloning to circumvent the risk of genetic disease or to promote particular traits, it is possible—perhaps likely—that new risks to the cloned child's health and fitness would be inadvertently introduced (including the forgoing of genetic novelty, a known asset in the constant struggle against microbial and parasitic diseases). Parental control is a double-edged sword, and proponents seem not to acknowledge the harms, both physical and psychological, that may befall the child whose genetic identity is selected in advance.

The case for cloning in the name of the child's health and well-being is certainly the strongest and most compelling. The desire that one's child be free from a given genetic disease is a worthy aspiration. We recognize there may be some unusual or extreme cases in which cloning might be the best means to serve this moral good, if other ethical obstacles could somehow be overcome. (A few of us also believe that the desire to give a child "improved" or "superior" genetic equipment is not necessarily to be condemned.) However, such aspirations could endanger the personal, familial, and societal goods supported by the character of human procreation. We are willing to grant that there may be exceptional cases in which cloning-to-produce-children is morally defensible; however, that being said, we would also argue that such cases do not justify the harmful experiments and social problems that might be entailed by engaging in human cloning. Hard cases are said to make bad law. The same would be true for succumbing to the rare, sentimentally appealing case in which cloning seems morally plausible.*

Finally, proponents do not adequately face up to the difficulty of how "well-being" is to be defined. Generally, they argue that these matters are to be left up to the free choices of parents and doctors. But this means that the judgments of "proper" and "improper" will be made according to subjective criteria alone, and under such circumstances, it will be almost impossible to rule out certain "improvements" as unacceptable.

In the sections that follow, we shall explain more fully why Members of the Council are not convinced by the arguments for cloning-to-produce-children, even in the most defensible cases. To see why this is so, we need to consider cloning-to-produce-children from the broadest possible moral perspective, beginning with ethical questions regarding experiments on human subjects. What we hope to show is that the frequently made safety arguments strike deeper than we usually realize, and that they point beyond themselves toward more fundamental moral objections to cloning-to-produce-children.

*   *   *

---

* Consider the following analogy: We would not allow a rare sympathetic case for brother-sister marriage—where, say, the two children were separated at birth and later fell in love, ignorant of their kinship—to overturn the taboo on incest. Whatever their merit, the goals of well-being and health do not outweigh the moral and social harms that cloning would entail.

II. The Case against Cloning-to-Produce-Children

A. The Ethics of Human Experimentation

We begin with concerns regarding the safety of the cloning procedure and the health of the participants. We do so for several reasons. First, these concerns are widely, indeed nearly unanimously, shared. Second, they lend themselves readily to familiar modes of ethical analysis—including concerns about harming the innocent, protecting human rights, and ensuring the consent of all research subjects. Finally, if carefully considered, these concerns begin to reveal the important ethical principles that must guide our broader assessment of cloning-to-produce-children. They suggest that human beings, unlike inanimate matter or even animals, are in some way *inviolable*, and therefore challenge us to reflect on what it is *about* human beings that makes them inviolable, and whether cloning-to-produce-children threatens these distinctly human goods.

In initiating this analysis, there is perhaps no better place to start than the long-standing international practice of regulating experiments on human subjects. After all, the cloning of a human being, as well as all the research and trials required before such a procedure could be expected to succeed, would constitute experiments on the individuals involved—the egg donor, the birthing mother, and especially the child-to-be. It therefore makes sense to consider the safety and health concerns that arise from cloning-to-produce-children in light of the widely shared ethical principles that govern experimentation on human subjects.

Since the Second World War, various codes for the ethical conduct of human experimentation have been adopted around the world. These codes and regulations were formulated in direct response to serious ethical lapses and violations committed by research scientists against the rights and dignity of individual human beings. Among the most important and widely accepted documents to emerge were the Nuremberg Code of 1947[7] and the Helsinki Declaration of 1964.[8] Influential in the United States is also the Belmont Report, published in 1978 by the National Commission for the Protection of Human Subjects of Biomedical and Behavioral Research.[9]

The Nuremberg Code laid out ten principles for the ethical conduct of experiments, focusing especially on voluntary consent of research subjects, the principle that experiments should be conducted only with the aim of providing a concrete good for society that is unprocurable by other methods, and with the avoidance of physical or mental harm. The Helsinki Declaration stated, among other things, that research should be undertaken only when the prospective benefit clearly outweighs the expected risk, when the research subject has been fully informed of all risks, and when the research-subject population is itself likely to benefit from the results of the experiment.

Finally, the Belmont Report proposed three basic ethical principles that were to guide the treatment of human subjects involved in scientific research. The first of these is *respect for persons*, which requires researchers to acknowledge the autonomy and individual rights of research subjects and to offer special protection to those with diminished autonomy and capacity. The second principle is *beneficence*. Scientific research must not only refrain from harming those involved but must also be aimed at helping them, or others, in concrete and important ways. The third principle is *justice*, which involves just distribution of potential benefits and harms and fair selection of research subjects. When applied, these general principles lead to both a requirement for informed consent of human research subjects and a requirement for a careful assessment of risks and benefits before proceeding with research. Safety, consent, and the rights of research subjects are thus given the highest priority.

It would be a mistake to view these codes in narrow or procedural terms, when in fact they embody society's profound sense that human beings are not to be treated as experimental guinea pigs for scientific research. Each of the codes was created to address a specific disaster involving research science—whether the experiments conducted by Nazi doctors on concentration camp prisoners, or the Willowbrook scandal in which mentally retarded children were infected with hepatitis, or the Tuskegee scandal in which underprivileged African-American men suffering from syphilis were observed but not treated by medical researchers—and each of the codes was an attempt to defend the inviolability and dignity of all human beings in the face of such threats and abuses. More simply stated, the codes attempt to defend the weak against the strong and to uphold the equal dignity of all human beings. In taking up the application of these codes to the case of cloning-to-produce-children, we would suggest that the proper approach is not simply to discover specific places where human cloning violates this or that stipulation of this or that code, but to grapple with how such cloning offends the spirit of these codes and what they seek to defend.

The ethics of research on human subjects suggest three sorts of problems that would arise in cloning-to-produce-children: (1) problems of safety; (2) a special problem of consent; and (3) problems of exploitation of women and the just distribution of risk. We shall consider each in turn.

1. Problems of Safety

First, cloning-to-produce-children is not now safe. Concerns about the safety of the individuals involved in a cloning procedure are shared by nearly everyone on all sides of the cloning debate. Even most proponents of cloning-to-produce-children generally qualify their support with a caveat about the safety of the procedure. Cloning experiments in other mammals strongly suggest that cloning-to-produce-children is, at least for now, far too risky to attempt.[10] Safety concerns revolve around potential dangers to the cloned child, as well as to the egg donor and the woman who would carry the cloned child to birth.

(a) Risks to the child. Risks to the cloned child-to-be must be taken especially seriously, both because they are most numerous and most serious and because—unlike the risks to the egg donor

and birth mother—they cannot be accepted knowingly and freely by the person who will bear them. In animal experiments to date, only a small percentage of implanted clones have resulted in live births, and a substantial portion of those live-born clones have suffered complications that proved fatal fairly quickly. Some serious though nonfatal abnormalities in cloned animals have also been observed, including substantially increased birth-size, liver and brain defects, and lung, kidney, and cardiovascular problems.[11]

Longer-term consequences are of course not known, as the oldest successfully cloned mammal is only six years of age. Medium-term consequences, including premature aging, immune system failure, and sudden unexplained death, have already become apparent in some cloned mammals. Some researchers have also expressed concerns that a donor nucleus from an individual who has lived for some years may have accumulated genetic mutations that—if the nucleus were used in the cloning of a new human life—may predispose the new individual to certain sorts of cancer and other diseases.[12]

(b) Risks to the egg donor and the birth mother. Accompanying the threats to the cloned child's health and well-being are risks to the health of the egg donors. These include risks to her future reproductive health caused by the hormonal treatments required for egg retrieval and general health risks resulting from the necessary superovulation.[13]

Animal studies also suggest the likelihood of health risks to the woman who carries the cloned fetus to term. The animal data suggest that late-term fetal losses and spontaneous abortions occur substantially more often with cloned fetuses than in natural pregnancies. In humans, such late-term fetal losses may lead to substantially increased maternal morbidity and mortality. In addition, animal studies have shown that many pregnancies involving cloned fetuses result in serious complications, including toxemia and excessive fluid accumulation in the uterus, both of which pose risks to the pregnant animal's health.[14] In one prominent cattle cloning study, just under one-third of the pregnant cows died from complications late in pregnancy.[15]

Reflecting on the dangers to birth mothers in animal cloning studies, the National Academy report concluded:

> Results of animal studies suggest that reproductive cloning of humans would similarly pose a high risk to the health of both fetus or infant and mother and lead to associated psychological risks for the mother as a consequence of late spontaneous abortions or the birth of a stillborn child or a child with severe health problems.[16]

(c) An abiding moral concern. Because of these risks, there is widespread agreement that, at least for now, attempts at cloning-to-produce-children would constitute unethical experimentation on human subjects and are therefore impermissible. These safety considerations were alone enough to lead the National Bioethics Advisory Commission in June 1997 to call for a temporary prohibition of human cloning-to-produce-children. Similar concerns, based on almost five more years of animal experimentation, convinced the panel of the National Academy of Sciences in January 2002 that the United States should ban such cloning for at least five years.

Past discussions of this subject have often given the impression that the safety concern is a purely temporary one that can be allayed in the near future, as scientific advances and improvements in technique reduce the risks to an ethically acceptable level. But this impression is mistaken, for considerable safety risks are likely to be enduring, perhaps permanent. If so, there will be abiding ethical difficulties *even with efforts aimed at making human cloning safe.*

The reason is clear: experiments to develop new reproductive technologies are necessarily intergenerational, undertaken to serve the reproductive desires of prospective parents but practiced also and always upon prospective children. Any such experiment unavoidably involves risks to the child-to-be, a being who is both the *product* and also the most vulnerable human *subject* of the research. Exposed to risk during the extremely sensitive life-shaping processes of his or her embryological development, any child-to-be is a singularly vulnerable creature, one maximally deserving of protection against risk of experimental (and other) harm. If experiments to learn how to clone a child are ever to be ethical, the degree of risk to that child-to-be would have to be extremely low, arguably no greater than for children-to-be who are conceived from union of egg and sperm. It is extremely unlikely that this moral burden can be met, not for decades if at all.

In multiple experiments involving six of the mammalian species cloned to date, more than 89 percent of the cloned embryos transferred to recipient females did not come to birth, and many of the live-born cloned animals are or become abnormal.[17] If success means achieving normal and healthy development not just at birth but throughout the life span, there is even less reason for confidence. The oldest cloned mammal (Dolly) is only six years old and has exhibited unusually early arthritis. The reasons for failure in animal cloning are not well understood. Also, no nonhuman primates have been cloned. It will be decades (at least) before we could obtain positive evidence that cloned primates might live a normal healthy (primate) life.

Even a high success rate in animals would not suffice by itself to make human trials morally acceptable. In addition to the usual uncertainties in jumping the gap from animal to human research, cloning is likely to present particularly difficult problems of interspecies difference. Animal experiments have already shown substantial differences in the reproductive success of identical cloning techniques used in different species.[18] If these results represent species-specific differences in, for example, the ease of epigenetic reprogramming and imprinting of the donor DNA, the magnitude of the risks to the child-to-be of the first human cloning experiments would be unknown and potentially large, no matter how much success had been achieved in animals. There can in principle be no direct experimental evidence sufficient for assessing the degree of such risk.*

Can a highly reduced risk of deformity, disease, and premature death in animal cloning, coupled with the inherently unpredictable risk of moving from animals to humans, ever be low enough to meet the ethically acceptable standard set by reproduction begun with egg and sperm? The answer, as a matter of necessity, can never be better than "Just possibly." Given the severity of the possible harms involved in human cloning, and given that those harms fall on the very vulnerable child-to-be, such an answer would seem to be enduringly inadequate.

Similar arguments, it is worth noting, were made before the first attempts at human in vitro fertilization. People suggested that it would be unethical experimentation even to try to determine whether IVF could be safely done. And then, of course, IVF was accomplished. Eventually, it became a common procedure, and today the moral argument about its safety seems to many people beside the point. Yet the fact of success in that case does not establish precedent in this one, nor does it mean that the first attempts at IVF were not in fact unethical experiments upon the unborn, despite the fortunate results.†

Be this as it may, the case of cloning is genuinely different. With IVF, assisted fertilization of egg by sperm immediately releases a

---

* It is of course true that there is always uncertainty about moving from animal to human experimentation or therapy. But in the usual case, what justifies the assumption of this added unknown risk is that the experimental subject is a likely beneficiary of the research, either directly or indirectly. And where this is not the case, risk may be assumed if there is informed and voluntary consent. Neither of these conditions applies for the child-to-be in human cloning experiments.

† Surprisingly, there has been very little systematic study of the offspring of in vitro fertilization. One recently published study has suggested that IVF (and especially intracytoplasmic sperm injection [ICSI]) may not be as benign as we had thought (Hansen, M., et al., "The Risk of Major Birth Defects after Intracytoplasmic Sperm Injection and In Vitro Fertilization," *New Eng. J. Med.* 346: 725-730, 2002).

developmental process, linked to the sexual union of the two gametes, that nature has selected over millions of years for the entire mammalian line. But in cloning experiments to produce children, researchers would be transforming a sexual system into an asexual one, a change that requires major and "unnatural" reprogramming of donor DNA if there is to be any chance of success. They are neither enabling nor restoring a natural process, and the alterations involved are such that success in one species cannot be presumed to predict success in another. Moreover, any new somatic mutations in the donor cell's chromosomal DNA would be passed along to the cloned child-to-be and its offspring. Here we can see even more the truly intergenerational character of cloning experimentation, and this should justify placing the highest moral burden of persuasion on those who would like to proceed with efforts to make cloning safe for producing children. (By reminding us of the need to protect the lives and well-being of our children and our children's children, this broader analysis of the safety question points toward larger moral objections to producing cloned children, objections that we shall consider shortly.)

It therefore appears to us that, given the dangers involved and the relatively limited goods to be gained from cloning-to-produce-children, conducting experiments in an effort to make cloning-to-produce-children safer would itself be an unacceptable violation of the norms of the ethics of research. *There seems to be no ethical way to try to discover whether cloning-to-produce-children can become safe, now or in the future.*

2. A Special Problem of Consent

A further concern relating to the ethics of human research revolves around the question of consent. Consent from the cloned child-to-be is of course impossible to obtain, and because no one consents to his or her own birth, it may be argued that concerns about consent are misplaced when applied to the unborn. But the issue is not so simple. For reasons having to do both with the safety concerns raised above and with the social, psychological, and moral concerns to be addressed below, an attempt to clone a human being would potentially expose a cloned individual-to-be to great risks of harm, quite distinct from those accompanying other sorts of reproduction. Given the risks, and the fact that consent cannot be obtained, the ethically correct choice may be to avoid the experiment. The fact that those engaged in cloning cannot ask an unconceived child for permission places a burden on the cloners, not on the child. Given that anyone considering creating a cloned child must know that he or she is putting a newly created human life at exceptional risk, the burden on the would-be cloners seems clear: they must make a compelling case why the procedure should not be avoided altogether.*

Reflections on the purpose and meaning of seeking consent support this point. Why, after all, does society insist upon consent as an essential principle of the ethics of scientific research? Along with honoring the free will of the subject, we insist on consent to protect the weak and the vulnerable, and in particular to protect them from the powerful. It would therefore be morally questionable, at the very least, to choose to impose potentially grave harm on an individual, especially in the very act of giving that individual life. Giving existence to a human being does not grant one the right to maim or harm that human being in research.

3. Problems of Exploitation of Women and Just Distribution of Risk

Cloning-to-produce-children may also lead to the exploitation of women who would be called upon to donate oocytes. Widespread use of the techniques of cloning-to-produce-children would require large numbers of eggs. Animal models suggest that several hundred eggs may be required before one attempt at cloning can be successful. The required oocytes would have to be donated, and the process of making them available would involve hormonal treatments to induce superovulation. If financial incentives are offered, they might lead poor women especially to

---

* The argument made in this paragraph is not unique to cloning. There may be other circumstances in which prospective parents, about to impose great risk of harm on a prospective child-to-be, might bear a comparable burden.

place themselves at risk in this way (and might also compromise the voluntariness of their "choice" to make donations). Thus, research on cloning-to-produce-children could impose disproportionate burdens on women, particularly low-income women.

4. Conclusion

These questions of the ethics of research—particularly the issue of physical safety—point clearly to the conclusion that cloning-to-produce-children is unacceptable. In reaching this conclusion, we join the National Bioethics Advisory Commission and the National Academy of Sciences. But we go beyond the findings of those distinguished bodies in also pointing to the dangers that will *always* be inherent in the very process of trying to make cloning-to-produce-children safer. On this ground, we conclude that the problem of safety is not a temporary ethical concern. It is rather an enduring moral concern that might not be surmountable and should thus preclude work toward the development of cloning techniques to produce children. In light of the risks and other ethical concerns raised by this form of human experimentation, *we therefore conclude that cloning-to-produce-children should not be attempted.*

For some people, the discussion of ethical objections to cloning-to-produce-children could end here. Our society's established codes and practices in regard to human experimentation by themselves offer compelling reasons to oppose indefinitely attempts to produce a human child by cloning. But there *is* more to be said.

First, many people who are repelled by or opposed to the prospect of cloning human beings are concerned not simply or primarily because the procedure is unsafe. To the contrary, their objection is to the use of a *perfected* cloning technology and to a society that would embrace or permit the production of cloned children. The ethical objection based on lack of safety is *not* really an objection to cloning *as such*. Indeed, it may in time become a vanishing objection should people be allowed to proceed—despite insuperable ethical objections such as the ones we have just offered—with experiments to perfect the technique.* Should this occur, the ethical assessment of cloning-to-produce-children would need to address itself to the merits (and demerits) of cloning itself, beyond the safety questions tied to the techniques used to produce cloned children. Thus, anticipating the possibility of a perfected and usable technology, it is important to delineate the case against the practice itself.

Moreover, because the Council is considering cloning within a broad context of present and projected techniques that can affect human procreation or alter the genetic makeup of our children, it is important that we consider the full range and depth of ethical issues raised by such efforts.

How should these issues be raised, and within what moral framework? Some, but by no means all, of the deepest moral concerns connected to human cloning could be handled by developing a richer consideration of the ethics of human experimentation. Usually—and regrettably—we apply the ethical principles governing research on human subjects in a utilitarian spirit, weighing benefits versus harms, and moreover using only a very narrow notion of "harm." The calculus that weighs benefits versus harms too often takes stock only of bodily harm or violations of patient autonomy, though some serious efforts have been made in recent years to consider broader issues. In addition, we often hold a rather narrow view of what constitutes "an experiment." Yet cloning-to-produce-children would be a "human experiment" in many senses, and risks of bodily harm and inadequate consent do not exhaust the ways in which cloning might do damage. As we have described, cloning-to-produce-children would be a *biological experiment*—with necessary uncertainties about the safety of the technique and the possibility of physical harm. But it would also be an *experiment in human procreation*—substituting asexual for sexual reproduction and treating children not as gifts but as our self-designed products. It

---

* Such improvements in technique could result in part from the practice of cloning-for-biomedical-research, were it to be allowed to go forward. This possibility is one of the issues we shall consider in evaluating the ethics of cloning-for-biomedical-research in Chapter Six.

would be an *experiment in human identity*—creating the first human beings to inherit a genetic identity lived in advance by another. It would be an *experiment in genetic choice and design*—producing the first children whose entire genetic makeup was selected in advance. It would be an *experiment in family and social life*—altering the relationships within the family and between the generations, for example, by turning "mothers" into "twin sisters" and "grandparents" into "parents," and by having children asymmetrically linked biologically to only one parent. And it would represent a *social experiment* for the entire society, insofar as the society accepted, even if only as a minority practice, this unprecedented and novel mode of producing our offspring.

By considering these other ways in which cloning would constitute an experiment, we could enlarge our analysis of the ethics of research with human subjects to assess possible *nonbodily* harms of cloning-to-produce-children. But valuable as this effort might be, we have not chosen to proceed in this way. Not all the important issues can be squeezed into the categories of harms and benefits. People can be mistreated or done an injustice whether they know it or not and quite apart from any experienced harm. Important human goods can be traduced, violated, or sacrificed without being registered in anyone's catalogue of harms. The form of bioethical inquiry we are attempting here will make every effort not to truncate the moral meaning of our actions and practices by placing them on the Procrustean bed of utilitarianism. To be sure, the ethical principles governing human research are highly useful in efforts to protect vulnerable individuals against the misconduct or indifference of the powerful. But a different frame of reference is needed to evaluate the human meaning of innovations that may affect the lives and humanity of everyone, vulnerable or not.

Of the arguments developed below, some are supported by most Council Members, while other arguments are shared by only some Members. Even among the arguments they share, different Members find different concerns to be weightier. Yet we all believe that the arguments presented in the sections that follow are worthy of consideration in the course of trying to assess *fully* the ethical issues involved. We have chosen to err on the side of inclusion rather than exclusion of arguments because we acknowledge that concerns now expressed by only a few may turn out in the future to be more important than those now shared by all. Our fuller assessment begins with an attempt to fathom the deepest meaning of human procreation and thus necessarily the meaning of raising children. Our analysis will then move onto questions dealing with the effects of cloning on individuals, family life, and society more generally.

B. The Human Context: Procreation and Child-Rearing

Were it to take place, cloning-to-produce-children would represent a challenge to the nature of human procreation and child-rearing. Cloning is, of course, not only a means of procreation. It is also a technology, a human experiment, and an exercise of freedom, among other things. But cloning would be most unusual, consequential, and most morally important as a new way of bringing children into the world and a new way of viewing their moral significance.

In Chapter One we outlined some morally significant features of human procreation and raised questions about how these would be altered by human cloning. We will now attempt to deepen that analysis, and begin with the salient fact that a child *is not made, but begotten.* Procreation is not making but the outgrowth of doing. A man and woman give themselves in love to each other, setting their projects aside in order to do just that. Yet a child results, arriving on its own, mysterious, independent, yet the fruit of the embrace.* Even were the child wished for, and consciously so, he or she is the issue of their love, not the product of their wills; the man and woman in no way produce or choose a *particular* child, as they might buy a particular car. Procreation can, of course, be assisted by human ingenuity (as with IVF). In such cases, it may become harder to see the child solely as a gift

---

* We are, of course, well aware that many children are conceived in casual, loveless, or even brutal acts of sexual intercourse, including rape and incest.

bestowed upon the parents' mutual self-giving and not to some degree as a product of their parental wills. Nonetheless, because it is still sexual reproduction, the children born with the help of IVF begin—as do all other children—with a certain genetic independence of their parents. They replicate neither their fathers nor their mothers, and this is a salutary reminder to parents of the independence they must one day grant their children and for which it is their duty to prepare them.

Gifts and blessings we learn to accept as gratefully as we can. Products of our wills we try to shape in accord with our desires. Procreation as traditionally understood invites acceptance, rather than reshaping, engineering, or designing the next generation. It invites us to accept limits to our control over the next generation. It invites us even—to put the point most strongly—to think of the child as one who is not simply our own, our possession. Certainly, it invites us to remember that the child does not exist simply for the happiness or fulfillment of the parents.

To be sure, parents do and must try to form and mold their children in various ways as they inure them to the demands of family life, prepare them for adulthood, and initiate them into the human community. But, even then, it is only our sense that these children are not our possessions that makes such parental nurture—which always threatens not to nourish but to stifle the child—safe.

This concern can be expressed not only in language about the relation between the generations but also in the language of equality. The things we make are not just like ourselves; they are the products of our wills, and their point and purpose are ours to determine. But a begotten child comes into the world just as its parents once did, and is therefore their equal in dignity and humanity.

The character of sexual procreation shapes the lives of children as well as parents. By giving rise to genetically new individuals, sexual reproduction imbues all human beings with a sense of individual identity and of occupying a place in this world that has never belonged to another. Our novel genetic identity symbolizes and foreshadows the unique, never-to-be-repeated character of each human life. At the same time, our emergence from the union of two individuals, themselves conceived and generated as we were, locates us immediately in a network of relation and natural affection.

Social identity, like genetic identity, is in significant measure tied to these biological facts. Societies around the world have structured social and economic responsibilities around the relationship between the generations established through sexual procreation, and have developed modes of child-rearing, family responsibility, and kinship behavior that revolve around the natural facts of begetting.

There is much more to be said about these matters, and they are vastly more complicated than we have indicated. There are, in addition, cultural differences in the way societies around the world regard the human significance of procreation or the way children are to be regarded and cared for. Yet we have said enough to indicate that the character and nature of human procreation matter deeply. They affect human life in endless subtle ways, and they shape families and communities. A proper regard for the profundity of human procreation (including child-rearing and parent-child relations) is, in our view, indispensable for a full assessment of the ethical implications of cloning-to-produce-children.

C. Identity, Manufacture, Eugenics, Family, and Society

Beyond the matter of procreation itself, we think it important to examine the possible psychological and emotional state of individuals produced by cloning, the well-being of their families, and the likely effects on society of permitting human cloning. These concerns would apply even if cloning-to-produce-children were conducted on a small scale; and they would apply in even the more innocent-seeming cloning scenarios, such as efforts to overcome infertility or to avoid the risk of genetic disease. Admittedly, these matters are necessarily speculative, for empirical evidence is lacking. Nevertheless, the importance of the various goods at stake justifies trying to think matters through in advance.

Keeping in mind our general observations about procreation, we proceed to examine a series of specific ethical issues and objections to cloning human children: (1) problems of identity and individuality; (2) concerns regarding manufacture; (3) the prospect of a new eugenics; (4) troubled family relations; and (5) effects on society.

1. Problems of Identity and Individuality

Cloning-to-produce-children could create serious problems of identity and individuality. This would be especially true if it were used to produce multiple "copies" of any single individual, as in one or another of the seemingly far-fetched futuristic scenarios in which cloning is often presented to the popular imagination. Yet questions of identity and individuality could arise even in small-scale cloning, even in the (supposedly) most innocent of cases, such as the production of a single cloned child within an intact family. Personal identity is, we would emphasize, a complex and subtle psychological phenomenon, shaped ultimately by the interaction of many diverse factors. But it does seem reasonably clear that cloning would at the very least present a unique and possibly disabling challenge to the formation of individual identity.

Cloned children may experience concerns about their distinctive identity not only because each will be genetically essentially identical to another human being, but also because they may resemble in appearance younger versions of the person who is their "father" or "mother." Of course, our genetic makeup does not by itself determine our identities. But our genetic uniqueness is an important source of our sense of who we are and how we regard ourselves. It is an emblem of independence and individuality. It endows us with a sense of life as a never-before-enacted possibility. Knowing and feeling that nobody has previously possessed our particular gift of natural characteristics, we go forward as genetically unique individuals into relatively indeterminate futures.

These new and unique genetic identities are rooted in the natural procreative process. A cloned child, by contrast, is at risk of living out a life overshadowed in important ways by the life of the "original"—general appearance being only the most obvious. Indeed, one of the reasons some people are interested in cloning is that the technique promises to produce in each case a particular individual whose traits and characteristics are already known. And however much or little one's genotype *actually* shapes one's natural capacities, it could mean a great deal to an individual's *experience* of life and the expectations that those who cloned him or her might have. The cloned child may be constantly compared to "the original," and may consciously or unconsciously hold himself or herself up to the genetic twin that came before. If the two individuals turned out to lead similar lives, the cloned person's achievements may be seen as derivative. If, as is perhaps more likely, the cloned person departed from the life of his or her progenitor, this very fact could be a source of constant scrutiny, especially in circumstances in which parents produced their cloned child to become something in particular. Living up to parental hopes and expectations is frequently a burden for children; it could be a far greater burden for a cloned individual. The shadow of the cloned child's "original" might be hard for the child to escape, as would parental attitudes that sought in the child's very existence to replicate, imitate, or replace the "original."

It may reasonably be argued that genetic individuality is not an indispensable human good, since identical twins share a common genotype and seem not to be harmed by it. But this argument misses the context and environment into which even a single human clone would be born. Identical twins have as progenitors two biological parents and are born together, before either one has developed and shown what his or her potential—natural or otherwise—may be. Each is largely free of the burden of measuring up to or even knowing in advance the genetic traits of the other, because both begin life together and neither is yet known to the world. But a clone is a genetic near-copy of a person who is already living or has already lived. This might constrain the clone's sense of self in ways that differ in kind from the experience of identical twins. Everything about the predecessor—from physical height and facial appearance, balding patterns and inherited diseases, to temperament and native talents, to shape of life and length of days, and even cause of death— will appear before the expectant eyes of the cloned person, always with at least the nagging concern that there, notwithstanding the grace of God, go I. The crucial matter, again, is not simply the truth regarding the extent to which genetic identity actually shapes us—though it surely does shape us to some extent. What matters is the cloned individual's *perception* of the significance of the "precedent life" and the way that perception cramps and limits a sense of self and independence.

2. Concerns regarding Manufacture

The likely impact of cloning on identity suggests an additional moral and social concern: the transformation of human procreation into human manufacture, of begetting into making. By using the terms "making" and "manufacture" we are not claiming that cloned children would be artifacts made altogether "by hand" or produced in factories. Rather, we are suggesting that they would, like other human "products," be brought into being in accordance with some pre-selected genetic pattern or design, and therefore in some sense "made to order" by their producers or progenitors.

Unlike natural procreation—or even most forms of assisted reproduction—cloning-to-produce-children would set out to create a child with a very particular genotype: namely, that of the somatic cell donor. Cloned children would thus be the first human beings whose entire genetic makeup is selected in advance. True, selection from among existing genotypes is not yet design of new ones. But the principle that would be established by human cloning is both far-reaching and completely novel: parents, with the help of science and technology, may determine in advance the genetic endowment of their children. To this point, parents have the right and the power to decide *whether* to have a child. With cloning, parents acquire the power, and presumably the right, to decide *what kind* of a child to have. Cloning would thus extend the power of one generation over the next—and the power of parents over their offspring—in ways that open the door, unintentionally or not, to a future project of genetic manipulation and genetic control.

Of course, there is no denying that we have already taken steps in the direction of such control. Preimplantation genetic diagnosis of embryos and prenatal diagnosis of fetuses—both now used to prevent the birth of individuals carrying genes for genetic diseases—reflect an only conditional acceptance of the next generation. With regard to *positive* selection for desired traits, some people already engage in the practice of sex selection, another example of conditional acceptance of offspring. But these precedents pale in comparison to the degree of control provided by cloning and, in any case, do not thereby provide a license to proceed with cloning. It is far from clear that it would be wise to proceed still farther in our attempts at control.

The problem with cloning-to-produce-children is not that artificial technique is used to assist reproduction. Neither is it that genes are being manipulated. We raise no objection to the use of the coming genetic technologies to treat individuals with genetic diseases, even in utero—though there would be issues regarding the protection of human subjects in research and the need to find boundaries between therapy and so-called enhancement (of this, more below). The problem has to do with the control of the entire genotype and the production of children to selected specifications.

Why does this matter? It matters because human dignity is at stake. In natural procreation, two individuals give life to a new human being whose endowments are not shaped deliberately by human will, whose being remains mysterious, and the open-endedness of whose future is ratified and embraced. Parents beget a child who enters the world exactly as they did—as an unmade gift, not as a product. Children born of this process stand equally beside their progenitors as fellow human beings, not beneath them as made objects. In this way, the uncontrolled beginnings of human procreation endow each new generation and each new individual with the dignity and freedom enjoyed by all who came before.

Most present forms of assisted reproduction imitate this natural process. While they do begin to introduce characteristics of manufacture and industrial technique, placing nascent human life for the first time in human hands, they do not control the final outcome. The end served by IVF is still the same as natural reproduction—the birth of a child from the union of gametes from two progenitors. Reproduction with the aid of such techniques still implicitly expresses a willingness to accept as a gift the product of a process we do not control. In IVF children emerge out of the same mysterious process from which their parents came, and are therefore not mere creatures of their parents.

By contrast, cloning-to-produce-children—and the forms of human manufacture it might make more possible in the future—seems quite different. Here, the process begins with a very specific final product in mind and would be tailored to produce that product. Even were cloning to be used solely to remedy infertility, the decision to clone the (sterile) father would be a decision, willy-nilly, that the child-to-be should be the near-twin of his "father." Anyone who would clone merely to ensure a "biologically related child" would be dictating a very specific form of biological relation: genetic virtual identity. In every case of cloning-to-produce-children, scientists or parents would set out to produce specific individuals for particular reasons. The procreative process could come to be seen increasingly as a means of meeting specific ends, and the resulting children would be products of a designed manufacturing process, products over whom we might think it proper to exercise "quality control." Even if, in any given case, we were to continue to think of the cloned child as a gift, *the act itself teaches a different lesson*, as the child becomes the continuation of a parental project. We would learn to receive the next generation less with gratitude and surprise than with control and mastery.

One possible result would be the industrialization and commercialization of human reproduction. Manufactured objects become commodities in the marketplace, and their manufacture comes to be guided by market principles and financial concerns. When the "products" are human beings, the "market" could become a profoundly dehumanizing force. Already there is commerce in egg donation for IVF, with ads offering large sums of money for egg donors with high SAT scores and particular physical features.

The concerns expressed here do not depend on cloning becoming a widespread practice. The introduction of the terms and ideas of production into the realm of human procreation would be troubling regardless of the scale involved; and the adoption of a market mentality in these matters could blind us to the deep moral character of bringing forth new life. Even were cloning children to be rare, the moral harms to a society that accepted it could be serious.

3. Prospect of a New Eugenics

For some of us, cloning-to-produce-children also raises concerns about the prospect of eugenics or, more modestly, about genetic "enhancement." We recognize that the term "eugenics" generally refers to attempts to improve the genetic constitution of a particular political community or of the human race through general policies such as population control, forced sterilization, directed mating, or the like. It does not ordinarily refer to actions of particular individuals attempting to improve the genetic endowment of their own descendants. Yet, although cloning does not in itself point to public policies by which the state would become involved in directing the development of the human gene pool, this might happen in illiberal regimes, like China, where the government already regulates procreation.* And, in liberal societies, cloning-to-produce-children could come to be used privately for individualized eugenic or "enhancement" purposes: in attempts to alter (with the aim of improving) the genetic constitution of one's own descendants—and, indirectly, of future generations.

Some people, in fact, see enhancement as the major purpose of cloning-to-produce-children. Those who favor eugenics and genetic enhancement were once far more open regarding their intentions to enable future generations to enjoy more advantageous genotypes. Toward these ends, they promoted the benefits of cloning: escape from the uncertain lottery of sex, controlled and humanly directed reproduction. In the present debate about cloning-to-produce-children, the case for eugenics and enhancement is not made openly, but it nonetheless remains an important motivation for some advocates. Should cloning-to-produce-children be introduced successfully, and should it turn out that the cloned humans do in fact inherit many of the natural talents of the "originals," some people may become interested in the prospects of using it to produce "enhanced children"—especially if other people's children were receiving comparable advantages.

Cloning can serve the ends of individualized enhancement either by avoiding the genetic defects that may arise when human reproduction is left to chance or by preserving and perpetuating outstanding genetic traits. In the future, if techniques of genetic enhancement through more precise genetic engineering became available, cloning could be useful for perpetuating the enhanced traits and for keeping any "superior" manmade genotype free of the flaws that sexual reproduction might otherwise introduce.

---

* According to official Chinese census figures for 2000, more than 116 male births were recorded for every 100 female births. It is generally believed that this is the result of the widespread use of prenatal sex selection and China's one-child policy, though it should be noted that even in a country such as South Korea, which has no such policy, the use of prenatal sex selection has skewed the sex ratio in favor of males.

"Private eugenics" does not carry with it the dark implications of state despotism or political control of the gene pool that characterized earlier eugenic proposals and the racist eugenic practices of the twentieth century. Nonetheless, it could prove dangerous to our humanity. Besides the dehumanizing prospects of the turn toward manufacture that such programs of enhancement would require, there is the further difficulty of the lack of standards to guide the choices for "improvement." To this point, biomedical technology has been applied to treating diseases in patients and has been governed, on the whole, by a commonsense view of health and disease. To be sure, there are differing views about how to define "health." And certain cosmetic, performance-enhancing, or hedonistic uses of biomedical techniques have already crossed any plausible boundary between therapy and enhancement, between healing the sick and "improving" our powers.* Yet, for the most part, it is by some commonsense views of health that we judge who is in need of medical treatment and what sort of treatment might be most appropriate. Even today's practice of a kind of "negative" eugenics—through prenatal genetic diagnosis and abortion of fetuses with certain genetic abnormalities—is informed by the desire to promote health.

The "positive" eugenics that could receive a great boost from human cloning, especially were it to be coupled with techniques of precise genetic modification, would not seek to restore sick human beings to natural health. Instead, it would seek to alter humanity, based upon subjective or arbitrary ideas of excellence. The effort may be guided by apparently good intentions: to improve the next generation and to enhance the quality of life of our descendants. But in the process of altering human nature, we would be abandoning the standard by which to judge the goodness or the wisdom of the particular aims. We would stand to lose the sense of what is and is not human.

The fear of a new eugenics is not, as is sometimes alleged, a concern born of some irrational fear of the future or the unknown.

---

* One thinks of certain forms of plastic surgery or recreational uses of euphoriant drugs, and the uses in athletics and schools of performance-enhancing drugs, such as anabolic steroids, erythropoietin, and Ritalin.

Neither is it born of hostility to technology or nostalgia for some premodern pseudo-golden age of superior naturalness. It is rather born of the rational recognition that once we move beyond therapy into efforts at enhancement, we are in uncharted waters without a map, without a compass, and without a clear destination that can tell us whether we are making improvements or the reverse. The time-honored and time-tested goods of human life, which we know to be good, would be put in jeopardy for the alleged and unknowable goods of a post-human future.

4. Troubled Family Relations

Cloning-to-produce-children could also prove damaging to family relations, despite the best of intentions. We do not assume that cloned children, once produced, would not be accepted, loved, or nurtured by their parents and relatives. On the contrary, we freely admit that, like any child, they might be welcomed into the cloning family. Nevertheless, the cloned child's place in the scheme of family relations might well be uncertain and confused. The usually clear designations of father and brother, mother and sister, would be confounded. A mother could give birth to her own genetic twin, and a father could be genetically virtually identical to his son. The cloned child's relation to his or her grandparents would span one and two generations at once. Every other family relation would be similarly confused. There is, of course, the valid counter-argument that holds that the "mother" could easily be defined as the person who gives birth to the child, regardless of the child's genetic origins, and for social purposes that may serve to eliminate some problems. But because of the special nature of cloning-to-produce-children, difficulties may be expected.

The crucial point is not the *absence* of the natural biological connections between parents and children. The crucial point is, on the contrary, the *presence* of a unique, one-sided, and replicative biological connection to only *one* progenitor. As a result, family relations involving cloning would differ from all existing family arrangements, including those formed through adoption or with the aid of IVF. A great many children, after all, are adopted, and live happy lives in loving families, in the absence of any biological connections with their parents. Children conceived by artificial insemination using donor sperm and by various IVF techniques may have unusual relationships with their genetic parents, or no genetic relationships at all. But all of these existing arrangements attempt in important ways to emulate the model of the natural family (at least in its arrangement of the generations), while cloning runs contrary to that model.

What the exact effects of cloning-to-produce-children might be for families is highly speculative, to be sure, but it is still worth flagging certain troubling possibilities and risks. The fact that the cloned child bears a special tie to only one parent may complicate family dynamics. As the child developed, it could not help but be regarded as specially akin to only one of his or her parents. The sins or failings of the father (or mother), if reappearing in the cloned child, might be blamed on the progenitor, adding to the chances of domestic turmoil. The problems of being and rearing an adolescent could become complicated should the teenage clone of the mother "reappear" as the double of the woman the father once fell in love with. Risks of competition, rivalry, jealousy, and parental tension could become heightened.*

Even if the child were cloned from someone who is not a member of the family in which the child is raised, the fact would remain that he or she has been produced in the nearly precise genetic image of another and for some particular reason, with some particular design in mind. Should this become known to the child, as most likely it would, a desire to seek out connection to the "original" could complicate his or her relation to the rearing family, as would living consciously "under the *reason*" for this extra-familial choice of progenitor. Though many people make

---

* And there might be special complications in the event of divorce. Does the child rightfully or more naturally belong to the "genetic parent"? How would a single parent deal with a child who shares none of her genes but carries 100 percent of the genes of the person she chose to divorce? Whether such foreseeable complications would in fact emerge is, of course, an empirical question that cannot be answered in advance. But knowledge of the complexities of family life lead us not to want to dismiss them.

light of the importance of biological kinship (compared to the bonds formed through rearing and experienced family life), many adopted children and children conceived by artificial insemination or IVF using donor sperm show by their actions that they do not agree. They make great efforts to locate their "biological parents," even where paternity consists in nothing more than the donation of sperm. Where the progenitor is a genetic near-twin, surely the urge of the cloned child to connect with the unknown "parent" would be still greater.

For all these reasons, the cloning family differs from the "natural family" or the "adoptive family." By breaking through the natural boundaries between generations, cloning could strain the social ties between them.

5. Effects on Society

The hazards and costs of cloning-to-produce-children may not be confined to the direct participants. The rest of society may also be at risk. The impact of human cloning on society at large may be the least appreciated, but among the most important, factors to consider in contemplating the morality of this activity.

Cloning is a human activity affecting not only those who are cloned or those who are clones, but also the entire society that allows or supports such activity. For insofar as the society *accepts* cloning-to-produce-children, to that extent the society may be said to *engage* in it. A society that allows dehumanizing practices—especially when given an opportunity to try to prevent them—risks becoming an accomplice in those practices. (The same could be said of a society that allowed even a few of its members to practice incest or polygamy.) Thus the question before us is whether cloning-to-produce-children is an activity that we, *as a society*, should engage in. In addressing this question, we must reach well beyond the rights of individuals and the difficulties or benefits that cloned children or their families might encounter. We must consider what kind of a society we wish to be, and, in particular, what forms of bringing children into the world we want to encourage and what sorts of relations between the generations we want to preserve.

Cloning-to-produce children could distort the way we raise and view children, by carrying to full expression many regrettable tendencies already present in our culture. We are already liable to regard children largely as vehicles for our own fulfillment and ambitions. The impulse to create "designer children" is present today—as temptation and social practice. The notion of life as a gift, mysterious and limited, is under siege. Cloning-to-produce-children would carry these tendencies and temptations to an extreme expression. It advances the notion that the child is but an object of our sovereign mastery.

A society that clones human beings thinks about human beings (and especially children) differently than does a society that refuses to do so. It could easily be argued that we have already in myriad ways begun to show signs of regarding our children as projects on which we may work our wills. Further, it could be argued that we have been so desensitized by our earlier steps in this direction that we do not recognize this tendency as a corruption. While some people contend that cloning-to-produce-children would not take us much further down a path we have already been traveling, we would emphasize that the precedent of treating children as projects cuts two ways in the moral argument. Instead of using this precedent to justify taking the next step of cloning, the next step might rather serve as a warning and a mirror in which we may discover reasons to reconsider what we are already doing. Precisely because the stakes are so high, precisely because the new biotechnologies touch not only our bodies and minds but also the very idea of our humanity, we should ask ourselves how we as a society want to approach questions of human dignity and flourishing.

D. Conclusion

Cloning-to-produce-children may represent a forerunner of what will be a growing number of capacities to intervene in and alter the human genetic endowment. No doubt, earlier human actions have produced changes in the human gene pool: to take only one example, the use of insulin to treat diabetics who otherwise would have died before reproducing has increased the genes for diabetes in the population. But different responsibilities accrue when one sets out to make such changes prospectively, directly, and deliberately. To do so without regard for the likelihood of serious unintended and unanticipated consequences would be the height of hubris. Systems of great complexity do not respond well to blunt human intervention, and one can hardly think of a more complex system—both natural and social—than that which surrounds human reproduction and the human genome. Given the enormous importance of what is at stake, we believe that the so-called "precautionary principle" should be our guide in this arena. This principle would suggest that scientists, technologists, and, indeed, all of us should be modest in claiming to understand the many possible consequences of any profound alteration of human procreation, especially where there are not compelling reasons to proceed. Lacking such understanding, no one should take action so drastic as the cloning of a human child. In the absence of the necessary human wisdom, prudence calls upon us to set limits on efforts to control and remake the character of human procreation and human life.

It is not only a matter of prudence. Cloning-to-produce-children would also be an *injustice* to the cloned child—from the imposition of the chromosomes of someone else, to the intentional deprivation of biological parents, to all of the possible bodily and psychological harms that we have enumerated in this chapter. It is ultimately the claim that the cloned child would be seriously wronged—and not only harmed in body—that would justify government intervention. It is to this question—the public policy question of what the government should and can do to prevent such injustice—that we will turn in Chapter Seven. But, regarding the ethical assessment, Members of the Council are in unanimous agreement that cloning-to-produce-children is not only unsafe but also morally unacceptable and ought not to be attempted.*

ENDNOTES

1 National Bioethics Advisory Commission, *Cloning Human Beings* Bethesda, MD, 1997.

2 National Academy of Sciences (NAS) *Scientific and Medical Aspects of Human Reproductive Cloning*, Washington, DC: National Academy Press, 2002. (Referred to in subsequent citations as NAS Report.)

3 NAS Report, pp. 6-7.

4 Lederberg, J. "Experimental Genetics and Human Evolution" *The American Naturalist*, September-October 1966.

5 Supreme Court of the United States. *Eisenstadt v. Baird*, 405 US 438, 1972.

6 Tribe, L. "On Not Banning Cloning for the Wrong Reasons" in Nussbaum, M., and C. R. Sunstein. *Clones and Clones: Facts and Fantasies about Human Cloning*. New York: Norton, 1998, p. 321.

7 Nuremberg Report. *Trials of War Criminals before the Nuremberg Military Tribunals under Control Council Law No. 10, Vol. 2, pp. 181-182.* Washington, DC: Government Printing Office, 1949.

8 Helsinki Declaration. 18th World Medical Association General Assembly *Ethical Principles for Medical Research Involving Human Subjects*, adopted in Helsinki, Finland, June 1964, and amended in October 1975, October 1983, September 1989, October 1996, and October 2000.

9 Belmont Report. The National Commission for the Protection of Human Subjects of Biomedical and Behavioral Research. *The Belmont Report: Ethical Principles and Guidelines for the Protection of Human Subjects of Research*. Bethesda, MD: Government Printing Office, 1978.

10 See, for instance, Chapter Four of the present report, as well as Chapter 3 of the NAS Report.

---

* Not surprisingly, some of us feel more strongly than others about this conclusion. One or two of us might someday be willing to see cloning-to-produce-children occur in the rare defensible case, but then only if means were available to confine its use to such cases.

[11] These issues are discussed in the NAS Report (3-2) as well as in Wilmut, I., Roslin Institute, Scotland. "Application of animal cloning data to human cloning," paper presented at *Workshop: Scientific and Medical Aspects of Human Cloning,* National Academy of Sciences, Washington, DC, August 7, 2001; and Hill, J., Cornell University. "Placental defects in nuclear transfer (cloned) animals," paper presented at *Workshop: Scientific and Medical Aspects of Human Cloning,* National Academy of Sciences, Washington, DC August 7, 2001.

[12] See, for instance, Chapter 3 of the NAS Report, and Kolata, G. "In Cloning, Failure Far Exceeds Success" *New York Times,* December 11, 2001, p. D1.

[13] See, for instance, Rimington, M., et al. "Counseling patients undergoing ovarian stimulation about the risks of ovarian hyper-stimulation syndrome." *Human Reproduction,* 14: 2921-2922, 1999; and Wakeley, K., and E. Grendys. "Reproductive technologies and risk of ovarian cancer." *Current Opinion in Obstetrics and Gynecology,* 12: 43-47, 2000.

[14] These issues are discussed in greater detail in Chapter 3 of the NAS Report.

[15] Hill J.R., et al. "Clinical and pathologic features of cloned transgenic calves and fetuses (13 case studies)" *Theriogenology* 8: 1451-1465, 1999.

[16] NAS Report, p. 3-2.

[17] NAS Report, Figure 3.

[18] See for instance the NAS Report, Appendix B, tables 1, 3, and 4.

Chapter Six

The Ethics of Cloning-for-Biomedical-Research

I. The Manner and Spirit of This Inquiry

The question of whether or not to proceed with human cloning-for-biomedical-research is a morally serious and difficult one. On the one hand, there is the promise that such research could lead to important knowledge of human embryological development and gene action, especially in cases in which there are genetic abnormalities that lead to disease. There is also the promise that such research could contribute to producing transplantable tissues and organs that could be effective in curing or reversing many dreaded illnesses and injuries—including Parkinson's disease, Alzheimer's disease, juvenile diabetes, and spinal cord injury. On the other hand, there are the morally relevant facts that this research involves the deliberate production, use, and ultimate destruction of cloned human embryos, and that the cloned embryos produced for research are no different from cloned embryos that could be used in attempts to produce cloned children. Complicating the moral assessment are questions about the likelihood that this research will deliver its promised benefits and about the possibility of equally promising, yet morally less problematic, approaches to the same scientific and medical goals. Finally, there is the ever-present danger of creating false hope among patients, and the risk of allowing the goodness of the end (finding cures for disease) to justify moral indifference to the means used to achieve it. Morally serious people may differ in their final judgment of the ethics of cloning-for-biomedical-research. But they do—or should—agree on this: that fidelity both to the highest moral and human aspirations of science and medicine and to the moral standards of the wider community requires that we consider not only why and how to proceed with new lines of research, but also whether there might be compelling reasons not to do so or certain limits that should be observed. Both the facts (scientific and moral) and our ethical principles must be consulted in trying to judge what is best.

Yet despite this general agreement, it is difficult to know how best to proceed in the present case. There are multiple questions about the right context for considering the ethics of cloning-for-biomedical-research. First, we must weigh whether to take up this matter in the context of deciding what to do about cloning-to-produce-children or in the somewhat different context of the ethics of embryo and stem cell research more generally. The issue has in fact emerged in the public moral debate over anti-cloning legislation, as a complication in the effort to stop cloning-to-produce-children. Generally speaking, the most effective way to prevent cloning-to-produce-children would arguably be to stop the process at the initial act of cloning, the production (by an act of somatic cell nuclear transfer [SCNT]) of the embryonic human clone. Yet such a measure would rule out cloning-for-biomedical-research, and many scientists and patient advocacy groups have argued that the human and moral costs of doing so are too great. Alternatively, we could take up this matter in what seems philosophically to be its more natural context, namely, as a sub-species of a larger inquiry into the ethics of embryo and stem cell research.

Each of these contexts—what to do about cloning-to-produce-children and what to do about embryo research—is certainly plausible. Yet each, by itself, is less than satisfactory. The first risks giving excessive weight to the fact that the embryos wanted for research are *cloned* embryos; the second, ignoring the aspect (central to cloning) of *genetic manipulation,* risks the opposite error by requiring that the ethics of cloning-for-biomedical-research be argued entirely in terms of what it is proper to do with *embryos as such.* We can imagine, in advance of any discussion, a variety of moral opinions that would emerge, influenced in part by how the question is formulated: one person could defend stem cell research performed using embryos produced by IVF but oppose research using cloned embryos for reasons of prudence (such as decreasing the likelihood of cloning-to-produce-children). Another person, holding IVF embryos in higher regard than cloned embryos, could reach precisely the opposite conclusion. Some people will hold that research on any human embryo, cloned or not, is always morally unacceptable (or acceptable), independent of whether ethical or legal guidelines are in place, while others will judge one way or another depending on whether appropriate guidelines and effective regulations have been established.

We have decided to discuss the ethics of cloning-for-biomedical-research in the broader moral-philosophical context, rather than the narrower moral-political one that has taken shape around the current debate over anti-cloning legislation. Though we are mindful of the importance of these public policy debates—and will consider them in the following chapter—we do not want our moral analysis to be skewed by the specific legal or policy questions at issue, especially as the moral questions discussed here have implications beyond the current political debate and even beyond the question of human cloning itself. We opt to take up the moral questions in their fullness.

A second question about context is even more difficult to assess. Should we regard cloning-for-biomedical-research as just the latest—and continuous—step in trying to unlock the secrets of human development and to discover cures for diseases? Or should it be seen—instead or also—as the earliest stage of a revolutionary new science of enhancement or eugenics, which will go beyond treating individuals with disease and disability to attempt engineered improvements in human genetic endowments? Because innovations like cloning come to us gradually and piecemeal, and because it cannot be known in advance how exactly they will be used or where they might lead, there is a temptation to stay close to the present and to ignore possible future implications.

Yet the alleged perils of going ahead with the research are arguably no more speculative than the promised benefits. And it would be morally and prudently shortsighted for this Council, charged with investigating "the human and moral significance of advances in biomedical science and technology," to refuse to think about where this research might lead. We will therefore consider, even if we cannot know in advance, whether and how the sort of genetic manipulation of embryos exemplified by cloning-for-biomedical-research is new or "revolutionary." Genetic therapy for existing diseases and non-therapeutic genetic modifications of our native endowments raise profoundly different questions. Accordingly, we will keep in sight not only the moral questions surrounding the *means* of cloning-for-biomedical-research—which is to say, the significance of using or not using nascent human life as a resource—but also the possible *ends* to which our expanding knowledge and capacities might be put. At the same time, we will be careful not to equate genetic medicine that is truly in the service of human life with genetic manipulation that is not, and to avoid both the unjustified fear and exaggerated promises that sometimes accompany biomedical progress.

A third difficulty concerns the relation between the ethics of research on embryos (cloned or not) and the ethics of abortion. For many people, these issues are linked, and there is doubtless an overlap in the moral questions involved. Yet the issues are, in important respects, quite distinct. In the case of abortion, the fetuses whose fate is at issue are unwanted and (usually) the result of unintended conception. The embryos produced for research are wanted, indeed deliberately created, with certain knowledge and intent that they will be used and destroyed. More important perhaps, the extra-corporeal embryo (whether produced specially for research or left-over in IVF procedures) does not exist in conflict with the wishes, interests, or rights of a woman who is pregnant. Also, although abortion is widely practiced, each decision to abort is made one at a time, case by case. In contrast, to embark on creating cloned embryos only for purposes of research is to countenance at one stroke the large-scale production of developing human life for routinized use and destruction. For these reasons, we shall try to consider the question of the ethics of research on embryos in its own terms, distinct from the ethical questions about abortion.

Finally, there is the question of the spirit in which this examination should be conducted. Reflecting the situation in American society, there are major differences within the Council regarding the morality of research involving early human (cloned) embryos. These differences turn largely, though not exclusively, on different judgments regarding the nature and moral status of the early human (cloned) embryo: namely, to what extent is it, or is it not, "one of us," a human life in process? Having explored these questions collegially among ourselves, we have come to think that *all* parties to this debate have something vital to defend, something vital not only to themselves but *also to their opponents in the debate*, and indeed to all human beings. No human being and no human society can afford to be callous to the needs of suffering humanity, cavalier regarding the treatment of nascent human life, or indifferent to the social effects of adopting in these matters one course of action rather than another.

We believe, therefore, that we can make our best contribution to a truthful and appropriate moral understanding of the issue by developing, in a single document, the moral cases both *for* and *against* proceeding with cloning-for-biomedical-research (and also articulating, where necessary and as clearly as possible, important differences within each of these cases). Each Member of the Council has been asked to help strengthen the case made for both sides, regardless of which side he or she inclines toward. By proceeding in this way, we hope to make clear to the President and the nation exactly what is morally and humanly at stake in the controversy and what may be gained *and lost* in whatever choice is finally made.

Thus, notwithstanding our differences, we stand together as the authors of the entire chapter, hoping by this means to shed light rather than heat on this most vexing of moral and policy questions. At the same time, we have tried fully and fairly to articulate our differences, and to do so by speaking, in the first person, as members of a deliberative body called upon to make our own best judgments. *This means that the "we" that now embraces all Members of the Council will stand in the particular sections presenting the moral case for and the moral case against cloning-for-biomedical-research (Parts III and IV, respectively),* **only** *for those among us who subscribe to the specific arguments being made in those sections. In other words, each opinion is a self-contained brief, representing not the Council as a whole but only a portion of the Council. And even within the cases for and against, Members of the Council disagree over matters of substance and emphasis.* But while the Council has strong differences of opinion, as delineated in the sections that follow, the Council speaks in a single voice in its affirmation that the debate must not be won by dismissing, ridiculing, or demonizing the other side. Important human goods are to be found on all sides of the debate, a fact too often overlooked.

We begin, in Part II, with a discussion of the human meaning of healing, for it is only by an analysis of this uniquely human activity that the contours of the debate over cloning-for-biomedical-research can be properly traced and understood. Here the Council speaks as one. What follows this framing discussion are two separate opinions: in Part III, a portion of Council Members make the moral case for biomedical research; in Part IV, a portion make the opposing moral case against. Going beyond just listing the arguments, pro and con, each opinion is a sustained attempt at moral suasion. Yet each opinion, by self-imposed stricture, has tried to respect and respond to the legitimate moral concerns of the other side and to indicate how it means to do them justice. Each has tried to address what is owed to embryonic human life, what is owed to suffering humanity, and what is owed to the moral well-being of society. This approach to public moral discourse is, we are well aware, an experiment. Whether it is successful or not is for the reader to judge.

*   *   *

II. The Human Meaning of Healing

Before presenting the two opinions, we will place the moral questions surrounding cloning-for-biomedical-research in their larger human context. Just as we did in discussing the ethics of cloning-to-produce-children, we step back from the particular technological possibility at hand to look carefully at the larger human goods that we seek both to serve and defend. We look specifically at the human meaning of healing the sick and aiding the suffering, as well as the spirit and practice of biomedical research that aims to make such healing possible. This exploration will better prepare us to see what is humanly at stake in our moral judgment about cloning-for-biomedical-research, and to face soberly both what is gained and what is lost in either proceeding or not proceeding. The subsequent moral arguments, both pro and con, are informed by these larger reflections.

To be human is to be mortal. To be alive is to be vulnerable to suffering. No one is better situated to appreciate these truths than the physician. To understand what it means to heal, one must therefore understand the doctor's special encounter with human suffering—as both an experience (a crying out) of the patient who lies before him and as a central mystery of human existence. Why do human beings suffer? Why do they suffer in ways that cannot be explained—entirely or perhaps at all—with human notions of justice? In this role, the doctor is sometimes a *messenger* of human finitude. He must tell patients that their days are numbered or that their time has come; he must tell grieving family members that death is at the door. But the healer is also and more importantly—in the eyes of both doctor and patient— a *deliverer*. Not only is he well armed to deliver us from specific maladies and miseries. He is also a much-needed ally against the deadly disease—traditionally regarded as a sin—of despair. Because of the moral aspirations of his calling, the physician is a trusted source of hope that the living might yet still live and that in his skill and the powerful techniques of modern medicine might lie the possibility of renewal. The doctor is, at different times, a reminder of the intractable sadness of human life, but also explicitly a conqueror who beats back suffering and disease with the saving hand of medical knowledge and technique, and who inspirits us with hope to go forward even in the absence of cure and relief.

Until roughly the second half of the twentieth century, physicians delivered more hope than cure, and they conquered few diseases. Since then, their arsenal against disease (at least in technologically advanced nations) has grown enormously, and it promises to grow greater in the decades ahead. New healing powers will surely emerge from the work of medicine's ally, biomedical research, firmly grounded in the principles and methods of modern biomedical science. This noble field of human endeavor also has a context in the larger domain of human life. Celebrating its achievements and eager for its gifts to human welfare, modern societies embrace and invest heavily in medical research and grant scientists great freedom to inquire and experiment. Because of the way science advances, freedom is crucial to the successful realization of its goals.

Dr. William Osler, one of the founding figures of modern medicine, described the aspirations of biomedical research as follows:

> To wrest from nature the secrets which have perplexed philosophers in all ages, to track to their sources the causes of disease, to correlate the vast stores of knowledge that they may be quickly available for the prevention and cure of disease—These are our ambitions.[1]

It is in the very nature of a "secret" that one cannot know in advance which areas of research and discovery will prove the most fruitful. One proceeds by trial and error. One makes hypotheses grounded in what is already known, in the effort to discover what remains a mystery. One begins with basic research into disease processes and mechanisms, in the hope that new knowledge will yield new medicines and new cures.

One motive for such research is simply the love of knowledge itself—the distinctively human desire to know, to see, to understand more than one already does. But biomedical research is also guided, above all, by the humanitarian desire to apply new knowledge in the service of those who suffer, to correlate knowledge that it "may be quickly available for the prevention and cure of disease." Biomedical scientists aim to weld the virtues of charity, beneficence, and responsibility to the human ambition to "wrest from nature" her secrets. This is the moral heart of both the medical profession and the research tradition that supports it: to do everything in our power, consistent with law and morals, to provide cures, amelioration, and relief to those who need them.

"Consistent with law and morals": this requirement qualifies "everything in our power." This limitation has been traditionally understood to be part of the healing vocation. Moral philosophers and philosophers of medicine have long held that the duty to heal is an "imperfect duty," meaning that it does not trump all other considerations. Physicians perhaps understand this best of all, learning their limits empirically from their encounters with patients whom they cannot save or even comfort. The duty to heal *this* patient, *at this time*, is also an imperfect one. After all, a cure for one person at the direct expense of another—for example, harvesting a vital organ from someone who is living to save someone else who is dying—would violate the first principle of medicine to "do no harm."

It is also true that scientific freedom and medical progress are not the only human goods worthy of our commitment and protection. Research must be judged both by the means it employs and by the ends it serves (both those that were intended and those that were not). The Nuremberg Code, the Helsinki Declaration, and the Belmont Report, discussed in the last chapter, are all efforts to set moral limits on biomedical research and to ensure that science serves human beings rather than the other way around. Among other things, these ethical codes embody the recognition that those who do research *about* human beings can never escape (nor should they) their status *as* human beings.

Those who investigate human biology are always both the *knowers* and *the subject that is known*, both the potential healers and the potentially afflicted. And therefore they must never treat that which is their equal—their fellow human beings—as something less than human.

But in the end, however imperfect it is as a duty and whatever its less than supreme place among all other human goods, the obligation to heal and to seek remedies is a powerful one. It is a mark both of man's natural limits (as the being in need of healing) and his capacity for goodness (as the being who heals). And so, the freedom of inquiry that makes biomedical research possible should be restricted only for the most important reasons, lest we do damage to the entire enterprise, or to the human beings and the society that benefit from the "vast stores of knowledge" it creates.

At the same time, however, those who have accepted the "healer's covenant"—and those who defend, engage in, and benefit from the research that improves and expands the human capacity to heal—must avoid the seduction of medical triumphalism: the belief that all human suffering, both physical and psychic, can be conquered by modern technique, and therefore that no form of biomedical research should be opposed. Doctors and scientists must not become partial human beings who evade moral responsibility by claiming that they are not qualified to judge the moral implications of their own medical research or, worse, that medically beneficial research is always self-justifying, and hence that there are no real moral dilemmas at all. In addition, they must avoid the cruelty of creating false hopes among patients and their loved ones, and the folly of creating messianic or utopian visions of what science and medicine can accomplish. And patients, even as they heroically fight against suffering, must not forget their own mortality—including the often unpredictable nature of how and when death comes.

These reflections point to the following conclusions: In judging the moral beneficence and moral hazards of medical research, we must remember that suffering should not be opposed by any means possible. We would be less than human if we did not desire to alleviate such suffering, but we would be imagining ourselves to be more than human if we thought and acted as if we could alleviate it once and for all. Rather, we must acknowledge that as human beings we live in a difficult "in-between." Whether as doctors, scientists, or as patients, we all wish for the possible renewal of life through medicine, but also acknowledge that suffering and mortality are part of being alive. We are morally obliged to seek relief of suffering, but only in ways that preserve our humanity.

With these realities in mind, this chapter will now take up the ethics of cloning-for-biomedical-research, and specifically the moral and human questions raised above: What is owed to those who suffer from debilitating injuries and diseases? What is owed to nascent human life? And what is owed to the moral well-being of society? These are the central questions in the debate, questions that Members of the Council over the past year struggled to answer, and that indeed every member of society must ponder when considering the ethics of cloning-for-biomedical-research.

* * *

A note about how the remainder of the chapter proceeds: Part III, delivered in the voice of some Members of the Council, makes the case for going forward with cloning-for-biomedical-research. Part IV, delivered in the voice of other Members of the Council, presents the opposing case, the argument against cloning-for-biomedical-research.

* * *

III. The Moral Case for Cloning-for-Biomedical-Research

The moral case for cloning-for-biomedical-research can be stated in the following straightforward way: American society and human communities in general have an obligation to try to heal the sick and relieve their suffering. This obligation, deeply rooted in the moral teaching of "love of neighbor," lies heaviest on physicians and health-care professionals who attend to individual patients. But it guides also the activities of biomedical scientists and biotechnologists whose pioneering research and discoveries provide new and better means of healing and relieving those who suffer. Research on cloned human embryos is one more path to discovering such means. Like embryonic stem cell research, to which it is partially related, it offers a promising approach to gaining knowledge and techniques that could lead to new treatments for chronic genetic or acquired degenerative diseases and disabilities.[2] If successful, it could help save countless human lives and ameliorate untold human suffering.

It is true that human cloning-for-biomedical-research raises ethical questions, mainly because it involves the production, use, and destruction of cloned human embryos. It is also true that cloned embryos produced for research could be used in attempts to produce cloned human children, and the availability of such cloned embryos for research and the perfection of cloning techniques might increase the likelihood that people will succeed in cloning children. We appreciate the concerns of people who voice these objections and risks, and we are prepared to accept certain limits and safeguards against possible abuses. Yet we believe that, on balance, the objections to cloning-for-biomedical-research are outweighed by the good that can be done for current and future individuals who suffer. The moral balance lies on the side of endorsing and encouraging this activity.

We who endorse cloning-for-biomedical-research will attempt to make a version of this case here. But we will do so, for the most part, in a somewhat different spirit, one that is informed by the discussion of healing just concluded. In moral debates about these matters, people often speak as if saving lives is the only value that counts and that everything else must be sacrificed to advancing potentially beneficial research. Others speak as if any failure to prevent death or suffering from disease is sinful. Our defense of cloning-for-biomedical-research is more complex and nuanced and, we believe, more true to the merits of the case in question. As we make our case, we will also confront—and accept—the burden of what it means to proceed with such research, just as those who oppose it must accept the burden of what it means not to proceed.

In making our case, we begin in Section A by summarizing the specific medical benefits that might be achieved by proceeding with this avenue of research. We then consider in Section B the moral dilemmas of this research. However, among those of us who believe the research should go forward there is disagreement about how seriously to take certain moral objections, and thus two distinct positions for proceeding are presented.

A. The Medical Promise of Cloning-for-Biomedical-Research

Many people suffer from chronic debilitating diseases and disabilities, including, among others, juvenile diabetes, Parkinson's disease, Alzheimer's disease, spinal cord injuries, heart disease, and amyotrophic lateral sclerosis. These terrible diseases shorten life, limit activity (often severely), and cause great suffering both for the afflicted and their families. The inspiring example of exceptional persons who bear bravely the great burdens of illness or injury should not blind us to the powerful warrants for research and therapy that might lift these burdens. The likelihood of premature death, in particular, can shadow the life of the patient and the patient's family even before it arrives, and its advent can impoverish and devastate families, dash hopes, and cast a chill on the lives of survivors. It is certainly admirable to confront, endure, and redeem these unchosen afflictions. But it is also admirable, where possible, to ameliorate through also admirable, where possible, to ameliorate through research and medicine the diseases and injuries that cause them.

Cloning-for-biomedical-research may offer unique ways of investigating and possibly treating several of these diseases. To unlock the secrets of a disease, scientists must explore its specific molecular and cellular mechanisms, carefully observing both normal and pathological development. This research could be greatly facilitated by in vitro cellular models of human disease. It is here that the potentially most valuable and unique benefits of research on cloned human embryos may lie. This section summarizes some of these benefits, with specific examples.

1. Cloning to Improve Understanding of Human Disease

The creation of cloned embryos using nuclei from individuals carrying genetic mutations—specifically, genes that predispose them to particular diseases—might be used to better understand and treat those diseases. Consider, for example, Parkinson's disease. A characteristic of Parkinson's disease is the aggregation in dying brain cells of a protein called alpha-synuclein. Two different mutations in the alpha-synuclein gene produce forms of the protein that aggregate more readily. Individuals carrying these gene mutations suffer from early-onset Parkinson's disease.

To study how genetic disease develops, scientists look for suitable laboratory models. One strategy for producing such disease models is to inject the disease-causing human genes into human or animal cells in tissue culture to produce a cell-system expressing the abnormality. Although it has been possible to introduce copies of mutant genes into various kinds of human and animal cells, the resulting in vitro cell-systems imperfectly model the human disease. In part this is because the behavior of specific proteins within cells is influenced by their interactions with other cellular proteins. For example, human alpha-synuclein in a mouse cell cytoplasm interacting with mouse proteins is unlikely to behave the same way that it does in a human cell surrounded by human proteins. To study human disease, it is generally preferable to work with human cells and tissues.

A preferable alternative to introducing mutant genes into normal cells is to begin with human cells that are already abnormal—in this case, cells carrying the mutant genes that predispose their bearers to Parkinson's disease. If one could obtain embryonic stem cells derived from cloned embryos produced using nuclei from individuals carrying these mutant genes, one could then stimulate them to differentiate into dopamine-producing nerve cells in vitro. These cells would provide a vastly improved model for understanding the metabolism of alpha-synuclein and its role in the development of Parkinson's disease.* In this example, the availability of improved in vitro models for genetic and neurodegenerative diseases could shorten the time required to understand them and to devise new treatments.

It is true that adult stem cells (or multipotent adult progenitor cells[3,4]), isolated from patients carrying the mutant genes that predispose them to Parkinson's disease, might also be stimulated to become dopamine-producing neurons in vitro. But there are unanswered questions about the ease of culture and long-term viability of such cells, and the likelihood of success with cellular models of disease derived from adult stem cells remains unknown. In the absence of a certain and superior alternative, it would be wrong to forgo the possibly unique benefits of cloning for disease research.

2. Cloning to Devise New Treatments for Human Diseases

The same cellular model systems used to study disease processes are also potentially useful for assessing and developing chemical or pharmaceutical treatments for the disease in question. To continue with the Parkinson's disease example, neurons derived from stem cells containing the alpha-synuclein aggregation muta-

---

* Once such cells were produced in one laboratory, they could be stored at low temperatures and supplied to other laboratories for study. And so, for at least this particular area of cloning-for-biomedical-research, it might not be necessary to perform the cloning experiment more than a few times for each disease, making it possible that the number of cloned embryos required will be limited.

tions would be very useful for testing compounds that might prevent aggregation of this protein. Chemicals that effectively prevented aggregation in this model system could be useful starting points for the development of new drugs for the specific treatment of Parkinson's disease. Here, too, neuronal cell-systems derived from adult stem cells carrying the mutations might serve as well as those derived from cloned embryonic stem cells. But there is no way of knowing in advance which of the alternative routes is more promising. From a medical and scientific point of view, research on cloned embryos may offer unique benefits.

3. Cloning to Produce Immune-Compatible Tissues for Transplantation

Some animal studies suggest that tissues derived from embryonic stem cells can, if injected under certain conditions, populate disease-stricken areas and differentiate so as to compensate for the loss of function caused by the diseased tissue. For example, liver or heart muscle cells injected into an animal with liver or heart disease could help regenerate the diseased tissues and restore normal function. But these cells would have a chance to do this only if they can survive the normal immunological rejection response to foreign material. Cloning-for-biomedical-research offers the possibility that scientists could someday generate individualized, "rejection-proof" replacement cells and tissues to help patients fight disease and restore health. Stem cells and tissues derived from an embryonic clone of the patient would have the same genes as the patient, and so, hypothetically, would not be rejected by the patient's body as foreign.

It is true that this possibility (what is sometimes called "therapeutic cloning") remains unproved.* As before, there may be alternative (nonembryonic or adult) sources of such "rejection-proof" stem cells and tissues derived from them. And there is ongoing research to circumvent the rejection problem altogether, by, for example, modifying the surface of an unrelated (embryonic) stem cell so as to enable it to escape detection as "foreign"

---

* See Chapter Four, in the section on stem cells and regenerative medicine.

tissue when transferred to patients for therapy. But, once again, it is too early to say which approach will work, and therefore it is important, from a medical and scientific perspective, not to close off any avenue of promise. The only way to verify this hypothesis is to try it—first in animals, then in human volunteers.

4. Cloning to Assist in Gene Therapy

Cloning techniques could also be combined with precise genetic manipulation to devise genetic treatments for genetic diseases. For example, a cloned embryo produced from a patient with severe combined immunodeficiency could be genetically modified to correct and repair the disease-causing mutation. Stem cells taken from the genetically modified cloned embryo might then be used to develop bone marrow stem cells to transplant back into the patient. This combined approach to gene therapy has shown early promise in one attempt to correct a genetic abnormality in the immune system of mice.[5]

B. Possible Moral Dilemmas of Proceeding

The potentially unique medical benefits of cloning-for-biomedical-research are, to those of us who favor it, abundantly clear. Yet the moral meaning of proceeding, still to be considered, is the subject of some debate among us. Most of us who favor proceeding believe that this area of promising research is nonetheless fraught with moral quandaries and ethical trade-offs; a minority of us do not share these concerns. The minority view, labeled Position Number Two, follows the principal moral case for cloning-for-biomedical-research under strict limits, designated here as Position Number One. Each opinion is presented in turn.

1. Position Number One

What makes this research morally controversial is that it involves the production, use, and intentional destruction of cloned human embryos. To determine whether or not the science should proceed—or, if it does, what limits should be placed on this research—it must be asked what, if anything, is owed this nascent form of human life. Only then can an evaluation be made of whether the possible benefits of this research justify its potential human cost. Other moral hazards must be considered that are either inherent in, or possible consequences of, this line of research. These hazards include the following: the possibility that cloned embryos will be developed and experimented upon beyond the blastocyst stage (the stage from which stem cells are taken); the possible exploitation of women who would be donors of eggs; the possibility that the production of cloned human embryos will lead—intentionally or unintentionally—to cloning-to-produce-children; and the possibility that engaging in such research will weaken or undermine society's respect for human life, and therefore undermine the very good (life) that it is meant to serve. Each of these moral challenges will now be addressed.

(a) What is owed to the cloned embryo? The subject of the moral status of developing human life is a difficult and controversial matter, one about which American society is and appears likely to remain deeply divided. We are well aware of the fact that we cannot do it full justice in the present context. Yet we believe that the moral defense of cloning-for-biomedical-research requires a consideration of what is owed nascent human life (cloned or not). There is also the question—considered at great length in Chapter Three—of whether cloned embryos are the moral equivalent of fertilized embryos, or whether the different nature of their origins and the uncertainty of their capacity to become full human beings means that our moral duties to them are somehow different.

Nevertheless, those who wish to defend cloning-for-biomedical-research—as we do here—must consider what is owed to *embryos as such* as well as the significance of the fact that the embryos in question would be *cloned*. That said, the relevant arguments, especially in this subsection and the next, are in most crucial respects the same as those regarding the treatment of embryos produced by IVF.

Let us be clear about what we are talking about when we speak of cloned *embryos*. We are talking about the very earliest stages in development, from the single cell product of SCNT, through the early cleavage stages, up to the blastocyst stage. This is a structure comprising some 100 to 200 cells not yet differentiated into specific tissues, let alone organs (though there is differentiation into inner cell mass and trophoblast; see Chapter Four). It is true that the embryos at the blastocyst stage, if implanted in a woman's uterus or (hypothetically) an animal or artificial womb, could be made to develop to later stages, and this potentiality must be taken into account. But it is important to keep in mind the primitive and undifferentiated condition of the embryonic stage that is relevant for the research in question.

We begin with a series of questions: Is destroying an embryo or cloned embryo at the blastocyst stage morally the same as killing a child? Is it the same as clipping a fingernail? Is it more like one of these acts than the other? Is it like neither? Does the moral status of an embryo depend on whether it is implanted in a woman's uterus or remains in a laboratory? Does the moral status of an embryo depend on its origins, or how it was produced? Does it depend on the motives of those who create it?

In our view, embryos have a developing and intermediate moral worth, such that the early human embryo has a moral status somewhere between that of ordinary human cells and that of a full human person. We acknowledge the difficulty of setting perfectly clear lines marking when an embryo's moral status goes from "less than a human person" to "like a human person" to "fully a human person." But we believe there are sound moral reasons for not regarding the embryo in its earliest stages (certainly in the first fourteen days) as the moral equivalent of a human person, though it does command significantly more respect than other human cells. We also hold that the embryo can be used for life-saving or potentially life-saving research while still being accorded the "special respect" it deserves, and while still preventing abuses such as research on later-stage embryos or fetuses or the production of cloned children. We will develop this view by taking up the significance of (i) twinning, (ii) implantation, (iii) the human form, and (iv) the notion of "special respect."

- *(i) The possibility of twinning.* First, it is still unclear in the initial fourteen-day period whether an embryo will develop into one or more human beings. The possibility for "twinning" is still present, suggesting that the earliest-stage embryo is either *not yet* an individual or is a being that is not confined to becoming *only one* individual. There are continuing philosophical debates about how to understand what happens in twinning: for example, whether one individual embryo "clones" itself to produce a second, or whether an organism that resembles (but is not *yet*) an individual embryo divides into two truly individual beings.* Nevertheless, the biological— and we believe moral—significance of the possibility for twinning is clear: after fourteen days (or after the primitive streak is formed), the being in question *can no longer be anything but a single being*—that is to say, no embryo after this stage, and thus no fetus or live-born baby, can replicate or divide to form another identical being. Before fourteen days, this possibility remains.

- *(ii) The moral significance of pregnancy and implantation.* Both IVF embryos and cloned embryos in vitro differ from comparable embryos conceived through sexual intercourse, for two reasons. First, the possibility for pregnancy with IVF or cloned embryos requires human assistance—that is, it requires the medical procedure of transferring an embryo into the woman's uterus. There is thus no possibility of the IVF or cloned embryo becoming a human child in its original in vitro environment. Second, embryos that are conceived through sexual intercourse have a direct physical connection with the individual women who carry them, whereas an in vitro embryo (cloned or not) has no such connection unless it is trans-

---

* In the first case, human individuality would be present from the start, in the second case, it would not, a morally significant distinction to some people.

ferred into a woman's uterus. Thus, transfer of cloned or IVF embryos into a woman's uterus is a significant moral step, insofar as such embryos cannot be removed—they can never again be held in human hands—without a direct physical intrusion or violation of the pregnant woman. Of course, it might become technologically possible in the future for in vitro embryos to develop beyond the blastocyst stage—and perhaps even to birth—without implantation into a woman's uterus (that is, in an artificial womb). Moreover, just because those embryos (cloned or not) that exist in vitro cannot continue to develop in a self-directed way beyond the blastocyst stage—that is, they require human artifice of some kind to develop further—does not mean that the preimplantation embryo is morally insignificant. But implantation does mark a significant point in these two respects: after implantation, self-direction toward birth (without external human artifice) becomes *possible* and external human control of embryos becomes *impossible* without intruding upon or violating the pregnant woman.

- *(iii) The significance of the developed human form.* Generally speaking, our moral sentiments respond very differently to the prospect—or the sight—of the destruction of an embryo and the murder of a child. In other words, there is a difference between *what we respect* and *what we consider inviolable.* The destruction of embryos might inspire concern or solemnity. In contrast, our reaction to the murder of a child would be one of horror, outrage, grief, and violation. James Q. Wilson has discussed how these two fundamentally different moral reactions change as the embryo develops into a fetus and then into a child—and correspondingly, how our concern and solemnity transform into horror and outrage.[6] Specifically, human beings exhibit a distinctly different moral sympathy for, and therefore greater willingness to protect, those organisms that have begun to resemble human beings in their developed form. The practice of sacrificing the life of the unborn in order to save the life of the pregnant woman—while not a moral parallel to the case of using cloned embryos for biomedical research—shows that there is some moral precedent for subordinating nascent human life to more developed human life. Of course, taken to an extreme, such a principle would justify the most grotesque uses of developing human fetuses for scientific experiments. Moreover, the case is not strictly analogous, for in the case of the pregnant woman, two lives are in conflict, a confrontation absent with free-standing embryos. We do not take the life of woman A's unborn fetus to save the life of woman B, not even with consent. But these difficulties notwithstanding, there is (again) a moral insight in this example. It demonstrates the important moral obligation of caring for those who already dwell among us, and the inevitable moral complexity of weighing different forms of human life, especially nascent and developed human life, against one another. It also suggests ways in which the claim on our protection may increase with the emergence of powers of awareness and suffering. Of course, such examples—and our moral sentiments in general—are not by themselves decisive. They are the beginning, not the end, of reasoning about our moral responsibilities. But they should also not be ignored for what they reveal about the nature of particular beings and particular acts—and in this case, for what they suggest about both the *developing* and *intermediate* status of the early human embryo.

- (iv) *The meaning of "special respect."* Finally, there is the question of whether it is possible to accord early-stage embryos "special respect" while still using them for biomedical research. We might reason here by an admittedly imperfect analogy. Various religions have rules governing the killing of animals for food. These exist in part to restrain cruelty. But they also serve to demonstrate respect for beings that command our affections and our wonder, because they are (like us) part of the mystery of existence. In a similar way, many hunters have a deep-rooted respect and even affection for the animals they kill. This is not to say that human embryos are the same as animals, because, in our opinion, they are indeed human organisms, if not fully developed human beings. But it is to show that there might be ways both to respect beings and to use them—for serious, not frivolous, reasons, and as part of our place in the order of being, not simply as an extension of our subjective will.

For the above-stated reasons, we would assign an intermediate and developing status to the human embryo. Those who treat the developing early embryo as nothing more than "mere cells" (see Position Number Two below) are in danger of ignoring its direct and inherent connection to the profound mystery of the origins of human life and seem willing to ignore the fact that an embryo will (and a cloned embryo might) eventually become one (or more) human being(s). This view greatly underestimates the moral seriousness of the question of whether to proceed with research on nascent human life. And it gravely mischaracterizes the meaning of potentiality—specifically, the difference between having the capacity to become anything at all (a pile of building materials, for example) and the capacity to become something in particular (an individuated human person or persons).

At the same time, those who believe that early-stage embryos are the moral equivalent of a human person (see Part IV below) are also, we believe, misguided. Just as we must listen to—and then articulate—the moral meaning of our disquiet at the idea of cloning-to-produce-children, we must listen to and articulate our fundamentally different moral responses to the destruction of an embryo on the one hand and the murder of a child on the other. While no single criterion like "appearance," "self-consciousness," "the capacity to express needs and desires," or "the capacity to feel pain" can by itself be decisive in conferring human dignity, the absence of all such criteria in the early-stage embryo or cloned embryo suggests that it is not a truly human being, but something different, commanding our respect because of what it is and may become, but yet not fully one of us.

In sum, what is owed the embryo is not the same protections, attachments, and rights as a human person; nor is it no respect at all. In making the decision to proceed with research on embryos or cloned embryos, we must do so only for the most compelling reasons—namely, the reasonable expectation that such research will save human lives—and only with eyes open to the moral burden of doing what we believe to be morally best. Even as we establish the biological and moral grounds for using human embryos in certain forms of research, we must face and accept the solemnity of what we propose. Finally, we must proceed with the paradox that accompanies all human suffering and human imperfection in full view: that sometimes we seem morally obligated to do morally troubling things, and that sometimes doing what is good means living with a heavy heart in doing it.

(b) The problem of deliberate creation for use in research. We next address whether the creation of embryos explicitly for the purposes of biomedical research presents additional ethical problems, beyond those just examined. In the case of research on cloned embryos, this form of deliberate production and destruction—rather than the use of leftover embryos initially created for reproductive purposes—is the only means of proceeding, if, at the same time, society prohibits cloning-to-produce-children. It is one thing to overcome the respect owed to an already existing embryo that would die even if not used for research. It is, some argue, quite another thing to bring the embryo into being solely for use and exploitation in research. Willing to accept the first, they reject the second.* In this connection, three issues seem worth considering.

First, the fundamental moral judgment about whether to proceed with cloning-for-biomedical-research must be grounded in

---

* See, for example, "The Ethics of Stem Cell Research," by Gene Outka, a paper presented and discussed at the Council's April 2002 meeting. Outka extends the principle "that nothing more be lost" to justify use of excess IVF embryos in research, but argues that this principle cannot be used to justify *creating* cloned (or IVF) embryos explicitly for research (available online at www.bioethics.gov). A slightly revised version has been published in the *Kennedy Institute of Ethics Journal* 12(2), 175-213, 2002.

our judgment about the moral status of the embryos themselves, not the purpose of their creation. If an embryo or a cloned embryo had no moral standing, then creation for research and eventual destruction would present no moral problem. If the embryo or cloned embryo were morally the equivalent of a child, then regardless of how or why it was produced, experiments upon it would be morally abhorrent. But if, as we have just argued, an embryo or a cloned embryo has a developing and intermediate moral status, certain worthy uses of them may be justified regardless of how and why they were produced. Because the use of stem cells from cloned embryos may in the future provide treatment for serious human diseases, the creation of cloned embryos and their subsequent disaggregation to isolate stem cells can be justified.

Second, the moral responsibilities for producing new embryos *solely* for research and for producing extra IVF embryos *later used* in research are not really so different. In the case of IVF and leftover embryos, the individuals who create them for reproductive purposes typically and deliberately create more embryos than they are likely to use, and therefore know in advance that some will probably be destroyed. It is true that they are produced with the intent of initiating a pregnancy and that the embryo wastage is not all that different from what obtains in efforts to conceive in vivo. But the moral responsibility for production, use, and destruction of leftover embryos are finally no less than for deliberate production for use (and subsequent destruction in research). (We acknowledge that some who accept this logic come to the opposite conclusion—namely, not that cloning-for-biomedical-research is morally permissible but that IVF should be morally restricted to creating one embryo at a time, if permitted at all.)

Third, in both cases—creating embryos to aid fertility or creating embryos for biomedical research—the ultimate goal is something humanly good: a child for an infertile couple or research that holds promise for curing debilitating diseases and easing suffering. Thus, in the case of cloning-for-biomedical-research, it is wrong to argue, as some do, that embryos are being "created for destruction." Certainly, their destruction is a known and un-avoidable effect, but the embryos are ultimately created for re-search in the service of life and medicine.

In the end, while we acknowledge the risk of turning nascent human life into a "resource"—fully separate from its intrinsic connection to human procreation—we hold that the concern over deliberate creation and destruction is misplaced. What matters instead is whether a proper regard is shown for the created embryos, and therefore whether a proper moral and legal framework can be established that limits and governs their use in accordance with the respect they are owed as *human* cloned embryos.

(c) Development and use of cloned embryos beyond the earliest stages. A perceived danger of allowing cloning-for-biomedical-research is that some researchers will develop cloned embryos beyond the blastocyst stage for research purposes. There are good scientific reasons and even moral arguments for doing so: one could learn much more about development, normal and abnormal, by going to later stages; and differentiated tissues taken from cloned fetuses would likely be more useful in regenerative medicine than stem cells. There is already at least one animal study showing the potential of this approach.[7] Transplantable functioning kidney tissue has been attained from six-week-old cloned cow fetuses, developed from cloned cow embryos transferred into a cow's uterus for partial gestation. Cloned human embryos might be developed past the blastocyst stage by implantation into an animal or human uterus, by the development of artificial wombs, or by advances in sustaining nascent human life in vitro.

This is a serious concern for those of us who believe that the cloned embryo has only an intermediate moral status and who also recognize the difficulty of drawing bright lines for when developing human life changes from "less than a human person" to "like a human person" to a "fully developed person." Clearly, the longer cloned embryos are allowed to develop, the more severe the moral burden in using them. And at some point, the moral burden of proceeding becomes a moral obligation not to proceed—even if significant medical benefits might be gained from doing so. In such circumstances, the medical principle of "do no harm" must override the researcher's desire to do good, lest we undermine the humanistic principles and spirit of the entire medical enterprise.

The moral tradition of "erecting a fence around the law"* may provide a useful guide in this case. We recommend that research on cloned embryos be strictly limited to the first fourteen days of development—a point just about when the primitive streak is formed and before organ differentiation occurs. We acknowledge that by erecting the fence more widely, we might be more certain to prevent this particular abuse (developing cloned embryos beyond the blastocyst stage). We also acknowledge that relaxing this limit to permit research beyond fourteen days might yield additional medical benefits. There is a moral burden in both directions. But we hold that there is a point of development beyond which research on nascent human life is morally intolerable no matter what the potential medical benefits. By raising a permanent fence at fourteen days, the dignity of human life will be sufficiently protected.

(d) Exploitation of women who are egg donors. Additional concerns in proceeding with cloning-for-biomedical-research are the possible dangers to, and exploitation of, women who are egg donors. The removal of eggs remains an unpleasant and (owing to the hormone treatments needed to hyperstimulate the ovaries) a risky medical procedure for women. It is therefore restricted mostly to circumstances where such a procedure is necessary to treat infertility—that is, where the women themselves are the beneficiaries of the procedure. Moreover, one possible avenue of cloning-for-biomedical-research—namely, the creation and future use of in-

---

* To increase the chances of keeping people from a serious transgression (the law), a prohibition is imposed (the fence) on activities that might lead or tempt one to commit it. For example, if the goal is to keep people from engaging in commerce on the Sabbath, one makes it unlawful for them to handle money on the Sabbath.

dividualized stem cells—would potentially require, if it became feasible, a very large and indefinite number of eggs.

These are genuine concerns. But they can be addressed by strictly adhering to the established body of ethics for research on human subjects. These ethical codes suggest the following requirements: regulation to prevent the creation of improper financial incentives for participating in such research; full disclosure by the users of human eggs of their practices; a commitment to consider using nonhuman eggs, so as to decrease the need for human egg donors*; and strict limits on the uses of cloned embryos for only those investigations that uniquely require them.

(e) The connection to cloning-to-produce-children. The final moral concern is that cloning-for-biomedical-research will lead—intentionally or not—to cloning-to-produce-children. For the reasons described in Chapter Five, we believe that the creation of cloned human children would be unethical and that society has a moral responsibility to ensure that this does not happen. Thus we are obliged to consider whether the pursuit of cloning-for-biomedical-research is consistent with a serious commitment to stopping cloning-to-produce-children. A number of points must be considered.

First, the production of cloned embryos, even for research purposes, crosses a new line by bringing into existence for the first time forms of nascent human life that are asexually produced. Second, experience with producing cloned embryos for biomedical research might well improve the technique of cloning itself, and therefore result in the greater perfection of the first step toward cloning-to-produce-children. Third, cloning-for-biomedical-research means that cloned embryos would exist in laboratories where they could be available for efforts to initiate a pregnancy. Finally, a society that allows cloning-for-biomedical-

---

* This means of reducing demand for human oocytes would imply increased SCNT of human nuclei into animal eggs, a practice that may bring additional moral questions. It was unanimously opposed by the National Institutes of Health Human Embryo Research Panel in its 1994 report (p. 82).

research, while setting strict legal limits on cloning-to-produce-children, will likely require the mandatory destruction of nascent human life.

The first concern is intrinsic to cloning-for-biomedical-research in itself. Are we a different society because we have brought asexually produced human embryos into existence? In some ways, perhaps we are. We are confronted by the scope of our powers to change human life, to alter human procreation, and to modify the nature of human origins and the genetic makeup of new life. But we are also reminded of what should be the animating purpose of that power: to cure disease and relieve suffering. We are reminded of both new and unique possibilities for human harm (from the production of human clones) and new and unique possibilities for human benefit (from research on cloned embryos). This is, we suggest, the meaning of crossing this line.

The second and third concerns are connected to where this research might lead: namely, to a perfected cloning technique and to the intentional production of cloned children. This is indeed a genuine concern. It is perhaps the case that the best way to prevent the production of cloned children is to prohibit the creation of cloned embryos. But in the end, we are not convinced that cloning-for-biomedical-research will inevitably lead to cloning-to-produce-children; rather, we believe that the best approach is a system of regulation that prevents such an abuse. Such a system would include: a legal ban on the implantation of cloned embryos in *any* uterus (human, animal, or artificial); a prohibition on developing cloned embryos beyond fourteen days; a requirement that any individual or group engaging in cloning-for-biomedical-research register with proper regulatory authorities; prior scientific review of all proposed uses of cloned embryos to judge their medical and scientific benefits; and strict accounting of all cloned embryos that are produced to prevent their removal from the lab of origin or their use in attempts at cloning-to-produce-children.

Of course, no system of regulation is perfect. There is always the possibility of malfeasance or error. The prudential question in this case is whether the likelihood of cloning-to-produce-children is increased—at all, slightly, or significantly—by allowing the production and use of cloned embryos for biomedical research. But there is also the question of whether some additional risk of cloning-to-produce-children is justified or tolerable given the human goods that might be achieved through cloning-for-biomedical-research. In our view, it is.

The final concern is that to pursue research on cloned embryos while preventing cloning-to-produce-children would require laws that mandated the destruction of nascent human life. In assessing the moral significance of this fact, we return to our judgment about the moral status of cloned embryos, what is owed to them, and whether the human goods that can be achieved by cloning-for-biomedical-research justify the real and potential human costs. In our view, the possible existence of a law requiring the destruction of cloned embryos at or before fourteen days of development would force moral clarity about what we are doing—and the burdens of doing it. Such a law might remind society of the ambiguity and limits of the efforts to "heal the world," and therefore the dangers of trying to do so by any means possible. The need for such a law requiring the destruction of nascent human life would also remind us that there is a burden in acting just as there is a burden in not acting.

(f) Conclusion. The case for cloning-for-biomedical-research—as with all research that involves the use of nascent human life—should not consist simply of guessing how many people might be saved and how many embryos might be lost. The moral concerns cannot so simply be taken up, addressed, and retired. They are permanent concerns and permanent burdens.

We believe, in this particular case, that the promise of cloning-for-biomedical-research justifies proceeding, but that the genuine possibility of moral harm requires strict regulations of how we proceed. We have tried to articulate what such a system of regulation might include: (1) a legal requirement not to develop cloned embryos beyond fourteen days of development and not to implant cloned embryos in any uterus, human, animal, or artificial; (2) the creation of a governmental oversight body to regulate individuals and groups who engage in this research, and to account for all cloned embryos that are produced so as to prevent their removal from the lab of origin or their use in cloning-to-produce-children; (3) a ban on commerce in living cloned human embryos; (4) adherence to the highest standards of the ethics of research on human subjects, especially when it comes to procuring eggs; (5) a prior scientific review of the proposed uses of cloned embryos to judge their unique medical and scientific benefits; and (6) continued research into possible non-embryonic sources of stem cells and tissues for developmental studies, and ways other than cloning to solve the immune rejection problem. Such regulations amount to much more than mere bureaucratic red tape. They embody a profound ethical insight—namely, that the means of serving human beings must never corrupt our responsibilities to human beings.

2. Position Number Two

A few of us who favor proceeding with cloning-for-biomedical-research have few of the ethical qualms expressed by our colleagues in Position Number One. It is our view that this research, at least in the forms and for the purposes presently contemplated, presents no special moral problems, and therefore should be endorsed with enthusiasm as a potential new means of gaining knowledge to serve humankind. Because we accord no special moral status to the early-stage cloned embryo, we believe that the moral issues involved in this research are no different from those that accompany many existing forms of biomedical research, requiring mainly the usual commitment to high standards for the quality of research, scientific integrity, and the need to obtain informed consent from, and to protect the health of, donors of the eggs and somatic cells used in nuclear transfer.

It is also our view that there are no sound reasons for treating the early-stage human embryo or cloned human embryo as anything special, or as having moral status greater than human somatic cells in tissue culture. A blastocyst (cloned or not), because it lacks any trace of a nervous system, has no capacity for suffering or conscious experience in any form—the special properties that, in our view, spell the difference between biological tissue and a human life worthy of respect and rights. Additional biological facts suggest that a blastocyst should not be identified with a unique individual person, even if the argument that it lacks sentience is set aside. A single blastocyst may, until the primitive streak is formed at around fourteen days, split into twins; conversely, two blastocysts may fuse to form a single (chimeric) organism. Moreover, most early-stage embryos that are produced naturally (that is, through the union of egg and sperm resulting from sexual intercourse) fail to implant and are therefore wasted or destroyed.

There is a moral precedent for using materials from early human embryos in the widely accepted practice of using organs from brain-dead human beings. Upon determination of death, and with permission from the next of kin, surgeons routinely harvest organs to save the lives of sick or dying patients. In a similar way, donors of somatic cells and human oocytes could justifiably grant a biomedical scientist permission to use cells derived from the resulting cloned five-to-six-day-old blastocyst, which also completely lacks a brain and a capacity for consciousness.

Some argue that the transplantation analogy is misleading, because a blastocyst has the potential to become a fetus and ultimately a child, whereas the brain-dead individual does not. But the *potential* to become something (or someone) is hardly the same as *being* something (or someone), any more than a pile of building materials is the same as a house. A cloned embryo's potential to become a human person can be realized, if at all, only by the further human act of implanting the cloned blastocyst into the uterus of a woman. Such implantation is not a part of cloning-for-biomedical-research, whose aims and actual practice do not require it.

Moreover, thanks to the results of nuclear transplantation research, there is reason to believe that every human cell has the genetic potential to develop into a complete human being, if used in cloning efforts to produce a child. If mere potentiality to develop into a human being is enough to make something morally human, then every human cell has a special or inviolable moral status, a view that is patently absurd.

"Slippery slope" warnings that the use of early-stage cloned embryos for research would lead necessarily either to the production of cloned children or to research on later-stage cloned fetuses should be treated with skepticism. Appropriate regulations can easily be established and enforced to prevent any such abuses. Although the continuity of biological development means that there is no naturally given moment after which an embryo or fetus becomes a person, defensible boundaries can be set. It is perfectly possible to treat a blastocyst as a clump of cells usable for lifesaving research, while prohibiting any such use of a later-stage embryo or fetus.

Where to set the boundary is a matter for prudent judgment. For the foreseeable future, the moral line might be safely drawn at fourteen days of development, when no nervous system has developed and when a distinct identity as a single individual has not yet been preordained. Also, derivation of the valuable stem cells can be accomplished well before fourteen days. Whether society will be faced, in the future, with reason to reconsider such a line is for now a matter of speculation. If such an occasion ever arose, it would require an evaluation of the proposed scientific use and its likely medical benefits and a moral consideration of whether the research in question justified using embryos beyond the fourteen-day point.

*   *   *

IV. The Moral Case against Cloning-for-Biomedical-Research

Our colleagues who joined in Part III in making the case for cloning-for-biomedical-research began their analysis by describing the medical promise of such research. Those of us who maintain—for both principled and prudential reasons—that cloning-for-biomedical-research *should not* be pursued similarly begin by acknowledging that substantial human goods might be gained from this research. Although it would be wrong to speak in ways that encourage false hope in those who are ill, as if a cure were likely in the near future, we who oppose such research take seriously its potential for one day yielding substantial (and perhaps unique) medical benefits. Even apart from more distant possibilities for advances in regenerative medicine, there are more immediate possibilities for progress in basic research and for developing models to study different diseases. All of us whose lives benefit enormously from medical advances that began with basic research know how great is our collective stake in continued scientific investigations. Only for very serious reasons—to avoid moral wrongdoing, to avoid harm to society, and to avoid foolish or unnecessary risks—should progress toward increased knowledge and advances that might relieve suffering or cure disease be slowed.

We also observe, however, that the realization of these medical benefits—like all speculative research and all wagers about the future—remains uncertain. There are grounds for questioning whether the proposed benefits of cloning-for-biomedical-research will be realized. And there may be other morally unproblematic ways to achieve similar scientific results and medical benefits. For example, promising results in research with non-embryonic and adult stem cells suggest that scientists may be able to make progress in regenerative medicine without engaging in cloning-for-biomedical-research. We can move forward with other, more developed forms of human stem cell research and with animal cloning. We can explore other routes for solving the immune rejection problem or to finding valuable cellular models of human disease.* Where such morally innocent alternatives exist, one could argue that the burden of persuasion lies on proponents to show not only that cloned embryo research is promising or desirable but that it is *necessary* to gain the sought-for medical benefits. Indeed, the Nuremberg Code of research ethics enunciates precisely this principle—that experimentation should be "such as to yield fruitful results for the good of society, *unprocurable by other methods or means of study.*" Because of all the scientific uncertainties—and the many possible avenues of research—that burden cannot at present be met.

But, we readily concede, these same uncertainties mean that no one—not the scientists, not the moralists, and not the patients whose suffering we all hope to ameliorate—can know for certain which avenues of research will prove most successful. Research using cloned embryos may in fact, as we said above, yield knowledge and benefits unobtainable by any other means.

With such possible benefits in view, what reasons could we have for saying "no" to cloning-for-biomedical-research? Why not leave this possible avenue of medical progress open? Why not put the cup to our lips? In *The Winter's Tale*, Shakespeare has Leontes, King of Silicia, explain why one might not.[8]

> There may be in the cup
> A spider steep'd, and one may drink, depart,
> And yet partake no venom, for his knowledge
> Is not infected; but if one present
> The abhorr'd ingredient to his eye, make known
> How he hath drunk, he cracks his gorge, his sides

---

* We are especially impressed by the promise of the research of Dr. Catherine Verfaillie and her group, showing the stability and multipotency of cells derived from bone marrow of animals and human adults. Should this work prove successful, it might serve all of the purposes said to require cells from *cloned* embryos. See presentation by Dr. Verfaillie at the April 25, 2002, meeting of the Council (transcript on the Council's website, www.bioethics.gov) and the papers cited in endnotes 3 and 4 to this chapter.

With violent hefts. I have drunk, and seen the spider.

To discern the spider in the cup is to see the moral reality of cloning-for-biomedical-research differently. It is to move beyond questions of immediately evident benefits or harms alone toward deeper questions about what an ongoing program of cloning-for-biomedical-research would mean.   In part, this approach compels us to think about embryo research generally, but cloning (even for research purposes alone) raises its own special concerns, since only cloned embryos could one day become cloned children. We need to consider and articulate the reasons why, despite the possibility of great benefits, society should nevertheless turn away and not drink from this cup, and why the reasons for "drinking with limits" (offered by our colleagues in Position Number One above) are finally not persuasive.

Our analysis proceeds along three pathways: what we owe to the embryo; what we owe to society; and what we owe to the suffering. We differ, among ourselves, on the relative importance of the various arguments presented below. But we all agree that *moral objections to the research itself* and *prudential considerations about where it is likely to lead* suggest that we should oppose cloning-for-biomedical-research, albeit with regret.

A. What We Owe to the Embryo

The embryo is, and perhaps will always be, something of a puzzle to us. In its rudimentary beginnings, it is so unlike the human beings we know and live with that it hardly seems to be one of us; yet, the fact of our own embryonic origin evokes in us respect for the wonder of emerging new human life. Even in the midst of much that is puzzling and uncertain, we would not want to lose that respect or ignore what we owe to the embryo.

The cell synthesized by somatic cell nuclear transfer, no less than the fertilized egg, is a human organism in its germinal stage.[*] It

---

[*] That the embryo in question is produced by cloning and not by the fertilization of an egg should not, in our view, lead us to treat it differently. The

is not just a "clump of cells" but an integrated, self-developing whole, capable (if all goes well) of the continued organic development characteristic of human beings. To be sure, the embryo does not yet have, except in potential, the full range of characteristics that distinguish the human species from others, but one need not have those characteristics in evidence in order to belong to the species. And of course human beings at some other stages of development—early in life, late in life, at any stage of life if severely disabled—do not forfeit their humanity simply for want of these distinguishing characteristics. We may observe different points in the life story of any human being—a beginning filled mostly with potential, a zenith at which the organism is in full flower, a decline in which only a residue remains of what is most distinctively human. But none of these points is itself the human being. That being is, rather, an organism with a continuous history. From zygote to irreversible coma, each human life is a single personal history.

But this fact still leaves unanswered the question of whether all stages of a human being's life have equal moral standing. Might there be sound biological or moral reasons for according the early-stage embryo only *partial* human worth or even none at all? If so, should such embryos be made available or even explicitly created for research that necessarily requires their destruction—especially if very real human good might come from it? Some of us who oppose cloning-for-biomedical-research hold that efforts to assign to the embryo a merely intermediate and developing moral status—that is, more humanly significant than other human cells, but less deserving of respect and protection than a human fetus or infant—are both biologically and morally unsustainable, and that the embryo is in fact fully "one of us": a human life in process, an equal member of the species *Homo sapiens* in the embryonic stage of his or her natural development. All of us who oppose going forward with cloning-for-biomedical-

---

cloned embryo is different in its origins, but not in its possible destiny, from a normal embryo. Were it brought to term it too would indisputably be a member of the human species. We caution against defining the cloned embryo into a "non-embryo"—especially when science provides no warrant for doing so.

research believe that it is incoherent and self-contradictory for our colleagues (in Position Number One) to claim that human embryos deserve "special respect" and to endorse nonetheless research that requires the creation, use, and destruction of these organisms, *especially when done routinely and on a large scale.*

The case for treating the early-stage embryo as simply the moral equivalent of all other human cells (Position Number Two, above) is entirely unconvincing: it denies the continuous history of human individuals from zygote to fetus to infant to child; it misunderstands the meaning of potentiality—and, specifically, the difference between a "being-on-the-way" (such as a developing human embryo) and a "pile of raw materials," which has no definite potential and which might become anything at all; and it ignores the hazardous moral precedent that the routinized creation, use, and destruction of nascent human life would establish for other areas of scientific research and social life.

The more serious questions are raised—about individuality, potentiality, and "special respect"—by those who assign an intermediate and developing moral status to the human embryo, and who believe that cloned embryos can be used (and destroyed) for biomedical research while still according them special human worth (Position Number One, above). But the arguments for this position—both biological and moral—are not convincing. For attempts to ground the special respect owed to a maturing embryo in certain of its developmental features do not succeed. And the invoking of a "special respect" owed to nascent human life seems to have little or no operative meaning once one sees what those who take this position are willing to countenance.

We are not persuaded by the argument that fourteen days marks a significant difference in moral status. Because the embryo's human and individual genetic identity is present from the start, nothing that happens later during the continuous development that follows—at fourteen days or any other time—is responsible for suddenly conferring a novel human individuality or identity. The scientific evidence suggests that the fourteen-day marker does not represent a biological event of moral significance;

rather, changes that occur at fourteen days are merely the visibly evident culmination of more subtle changes that have taken place earlier and that are driving the organism toward maturity. Indeed, many advocates of cloning-for-biomedical-research implicitly recognize the arbitrariness of the fourteen-day line. The medical benefits to be gained by conducting research beyond the fourteen-day line are widely appreciated, and some people have already hinted that this supposed moral and biological boundary can be moved should the medical benefits warrant doing so (see Position Number Two, above).

There are also problems with the claim that its capacity for "twinning" proves that the early embryo is not yet an individual or that the embryo's moral status is more significant after the capacity for twinning is gone. There is the obvious rejoinder that if one locus of moral status can become two, its moral standing does not thereby diminish but rather increases. More specifically, the possibility of twinning does not rebut the individuality of the early embryo from its beginning. The fact that where "John" alone once was there are now both "John" and "Jim" does not call into question the presence of "John" at the outset. Hence, we need not doubt that even the earliest cloned embryo is an individual human organism in its germinal stage. Its capacity for twinning may simply be one of the characteristic capacities of an individual human organism at that particular stage of development, just as the capacity for crawling, walking, and running, or cooing, babbling, and speaking are capacities that are also unique to particular stages of human development. Alternatively, from a developmental science perspective, twinning may not turn out to be an intrinsic process within embryogenesis. Rather, it may be a response to a disruption of normal development from which the embryo recovers and then forms two. Twinning would thus be a testament to the resilience of self-regulation and compensatory repair within early life, not the lack of individuation in the early embryo. From this perspective, twinning is further testimony to the potency of the individual (in this case two) to fullness of form.

We are also not persuaded by the claim that in vitro embryos (whether created through IVF or cloning) have a lesser moral status than embryos that have been implanted into a woman's uterus, because they cannot develop without further human assistance. The suggestion that extra-corporeal embryos are not yet individual human organisms-on-the-way, but rather special human cells that acquire only through implantation the potential to become individual human organisms-on-the-way, rests on a misunderstanding of the meaning and significance of potentiality. An embryo is, by definition and by its nature, potentially a fully developed human person; its potential for maturation is a characteristic it *actually* has, and from the start. The fact that embryos have been created outside their natural environment—which is to say, outside the woman's body—and are therefore limited in their ability to realize their natural capacities, does not affect either the potential or the moral status of the beings themselves. A bird forced to live in a cage its entire life may never learn to fly. But this does not mean it is less of a bird, or that it lacks the immanent potentiality to fly on feathered wings. It means only that a caged bird—like an in vitro human embryo—has been deprived of its proper environment. There may, of course, be good human reasons to create embryos outside their natural environments—most obviously, to aid infertile couples. But doing so does not obliterate the moral status of the embryos themselves.

As we have noted, many proponents of cloning-for-biomedical-research (and for embryo research more generally) do not deny that we owe the human embryo special moral respect. Indeed, they have wanted positively to affirm it.* But we do not under-

---

* Thus, for example, the 1994 report of the National Institutes of Health Human Embryo Research Panel, even while endorsing embryo research under certain circumstances, spoke (p. xi) of "respect for the special character of the preimplantation human embryo" and affirmed (p. x) that "the preimplantation human embryo warrants serious moral consideration as a developing form of human life" (though not, the report added, "the same moral status as infants and children"). Another report, *Ethical Issues in Human Stem Cell Research*, released in 1999 by the National Bioethics Advisory Commission, while declining to claim that the embryo should receive "the same level of respect accorded persons" (p. 50), spoke of and seemed to endorse the "ethical intui-

stand what it means to claim that one is treating cloned embryos with special respect when one decides to create them intentionally for research that necessarily leads to their destruction. This respect is allegedly demonstrated by limiting such research—and therefore limiting the numbers of embryos that may be created, used, and destroyed—to only the most serious purposes: namely, scientific investigations that hold out the potential for curing diseases or relieving suffering. But this self-limitation shows only that our purposes are steadfastly high-minded; it does not show that the *means* of pursuing these purposes are *respectful of the cloned embryos* that are necessarily violated, exploited, and destroyed in the process. To the contrary, a true respect for a being would nurture and encourage it toward its own flourishing.

It is, of course, possible to have reverence for a life that one kills. This is memorably displayed, for example, by the fisherman Santiago in Ernest Hemingway's *The Old Man and the Sea*, who wonders whether it is a sin to kill fish even if doing so would feed hungry people. But it seems difficult to claim—even in theory but especially in practice—the presence of reverence once we run a stockyard or raise calves for veal—that is, once we treat the animals we kill (as we often do) simply as resources or commodities. In a similar way, we find it difficult to imagine that bio-technology companies or scientists who routinely engaged in cloning-for-biomedical-research would evince solemn respect for human life each time a cloned embryo was used and destroyed. Things we exploit even occasionally tend to lose their special value. It seems scarcely possible to preserve a spirit of humility and solemnity while engaging in routinized (and in many cases corporately competitive) research that creates, uses, and destroys them.

The mystery that surrounds the human embryo is undeniable. But so is the fact that each human person began as an embryo, and that this embryo, once formed, had the unique potential to become a unique human person. This is the meaning of our em-

tion" that "the act of creating an embryo for reproduction is respectful in a way that is commensurate with the moral status of embryos, while the act of creating an embryo for research is not" (p. 56).

bodied condition and the biology that describes it. If we add to this description a commitment to equal treatment—the moral principle that every human life deserves our equal respect—we begin to see how difficult it must be to suggest that a human embryo, even in its most undeveloped and germinal stage, could simply be used for the good of others and then destroyed. Justifying our intention of using (and destroying) human embryos for the purpose of biomedical research would force us either to ignore the truth of our own continuing personal histories from their beginning in embryonic life or to weaken the commitment to human equality that has been so slowly and laboriously developed in our cultural history.

Equal treatment of human beings does not, of course, mean identical treatment, as all parents know who have more than one child. And from one perspective, the fact that the embryo seems to amount to so little—seems to be little more than a clump of cells—invites us to suppose that its claims upon us can also not amount to much. We are, many have noted, likely to grieve the death of an embryo less than the death of a newborn child. But, then, we are also likely to grieve the death of an eighty-five-year-old father less than the death of a forty-five-year-old father. Perhaps, even, we may grieve the death of a newborn child less than the death of a twelve-year-old. We might grieve differently at the death of a healthy eighty-year-old than at the death of a severely demented eighty-year-old. Put differently, we might note how even the researcher in the laboratory may react with excitement and anticipation as cell division begins. Thus, reproductive physiologist Robert Edwards, who, together with Dr. Patrick Steptoe, helped produce Louise Brown, the first "test-tube baby," said of her: "The last time I saw her, she was just eight cells in a test-tube. She was beautiful then, and she's still beautiful now."[9] The embryo seems to amount to little; yet it has the capacity to become what to all of us seems very much indeed. There is a trajectory to the life story of human beings, and it is inevitable—and appropriate—that our emotional responses should be different at different points in that trajectory. Nevertheless, these emotions, quite naturally and appropriately different, would be misused if we calibrated the degree of respect we owe each other on the basis of such responses. In fact, we are obligated to try to shape and form our emotional responses—and our moral sentiments—so that they are more in accord with the moral respect we owe to those whose capacities are least developed (or those whom society may have wrongly defined as "non-persons" or "nonentities").

In short, how we respond to the weakest among us, to those who are nowhere near the zenith of human flourishing, says much about our willingness to envision the boundaries of humanity expansively and inclusively. It challenges—in the face of what we can know and what we cannot know about the human embryo—the depth of our commitment to equality. If from one perspective the fact that the embryo seems to amount to little may invite a weakening of our respect, from another perspective its seeming insignificance should awaken in us a sense of shared humanity. This was once our own condition. From origins that seem so little came our kin, our friends, our fellow citizens, and all human beings, whether known to us or not. In fact, precisely because the embryo seems to amount to so little, our responsibility to respect and protect its life correspondingly increases. As Hans Jonas once remarked, a true humanism would recognize "the inflexible principle that utter helplessness demands utter protection."[10]

B. What We Owe to Society

Having acknowledged all that, we would miss something if we stopped with what is owed to the embryo—with the language of respect, claims, or rights. An embryo may seem to amount to little or nothing, but that very insignificance tests not the embryo's humanity but our own. Even those who are uncertain about the precise moral status of the human embryo—indeed, even those who believe that it has only intermediate and developing status—have sound ethical-prudential reasons to refrain from using embryos for utilitarian purposes. Moreover, when the embryos to be used have been produced by cloning, there are additional moral dilemmas that go beyond the ethics of embryo research alone. There are principled reasons why people who *accept* research on leftover IVF embryos created initially for reproductive purposes should *oppose* the creation and use of cloned embryos explicitly for research. And there are powerful reasons to worry about where this research will lead us. All these objections have their ground not only in the embryo's character but also in our own, and in concern not only for the fate of nascent human life but for the moral well-being of society as a whole. *One need not believe the embryo is fully human to object vigorously to cloning-for-biomedical-research.*

We are concerned especially about three ways in which giving our moral approval to such research would harm the character of our common life and the way of life we want to transmit to future generations: (i) by crossing the boundary from sexual to asexual reproduction, in the process approving, whether recognized or not, genetic manipulation and control of nascent human life; (ii) by allowing and endorsing the complete instrumentalization of human embryos; and (iii) by opening the door to other—for some of us, far greater—moral hazards, such as cloning-to-produce-children or research on later-stage human embryos and fetuses.

1. Asexual Reproduction and the Genetic Manipulation of Embryos

It is worth noting that human cloning—including cloning-for-biomedical-research itself and not simply cloning-to-produce-children—would cross a natural boundary between sexual and asexual reproduction, reducing the likelihood that we could either retrace our steps or keep from taking further steps. Cloning-for-biomedical-research and cloning-to-produce-children both begin with the same act of cloning: the production of a human embryo that is genetically virtually identical to its progenitor. The cloned embryo would therefore be the first human organism with a single genetic "parent" and, equally important, with a genetic constitution that is known and selected in advance. Both uses of cloning mark a significant leap in human power and human control over our genetic origins. Both involve deliberate genetic manipulation of nascent human life. It is, of course, precisely this genetic control that makes cloned embryos uniquely appealing and perhaps uniquely useful to those who seek to conduct research on them. But we should not be deceived about what we are agreeing to if we agree to start to clone: saying yes to cloned embryos in laboratories means saying yes *in principle* to an ever-expanding genetic mastery of one generation over the next.

2. The Complete Instrumentalization of Nascent Human Life

By approving the production of cloned embryos for the sole purpose of research, society would transgress yet another moral boundary: that separating the different ways in which embryos might become available for human experimentation. It is one thing, as some have argued, to conduct research on leftover embryos from IVF procedures, which were created in attempts to have a child and, once no longer needed or wanted, are "destined" for destruction in any case. It is quite another to create embryos *solely* for research that will unavoidably and necessarily destroy them. Thus, for example, the National Bioethics Advisory Commission (in its report on stem cell research) reasoned that in circumstances where embryos were going to be discarded anyway, it did not undermine the moral respect owed to them if they were destroyed in one way (through research) rather than another (by being discarded when no longer wanted for IVF).[11] By contrast, the Commission reasoned that it was much harder to embrace the language of respect for the embryo if it were produced solely for purposes of research and, having been used, then destroyed. This argument maintained the following moral and practical distinction: that embryos created for reproduction but no longer desired could, with proper consent, be used as research subjects, but that embryos ought not be produced solely in order to be used as research subjects. So long as we oppose morally and may perhaps one day prohibit legally the production of cloned children, it is in the very nature of the case that cloned human embryos will not be acquirable as "spare" embryos left over from attempts at reproduction. To the contrary, they will have to be produced solely and explicitly for the purpose of biomedical research, with no other end in view.

Some have argued that there is no significant moral difference between creating excess IVF embryos for reproduction *knowing in advance* that some will be discarded and creating cloned embryos for research *that leads necessarily* to their destruction. Because in both cases embryos are wittingly destroyed, there is, so the argument goes, no moral difference here.

When viewed simply in terms of the fates of embryos once they are created, the distinction between using leftover embryos and creating embryos solely for research may indeed be morally insignificant. But when viewed in terms of the different effects these two activities might have on the moral fabric of society—and the different moral dispositions of those who decide to produce embryos for these different purposes—the issue is more complex. In the eyes of those who create IVF embryos to produce a child, *every embryo*, at the moment of its creation, is *a potential child*. Even though more eggs are fertilized than will be transferred to a woman, each embryo is brought into being as an end in itself, not simply as a means to other ends. Precisely because one cannot tell which IVF embryo is going to reach the blastocyst stage, implant itself in the uterine wall, and develop into a child, the embryo "wastage" in IVF is more analogous to the embryo wastage in natural sexual intercourse practiced by a couple trying to get pregnant than it is to the creation and use of embryos that requires (without exception) their destruction.

Those who minimize or deny this distinction—between producing embryos hoping that one of them will become a child and producing embryos so that they can be used (and destroyed) in research—demonstrate the very problem we are worried about. Having become comfortable with seeing embryos as a means to noble ends (be it having a child or conducting biomedical research), they have lost sight of the fact that the embryos that we create as potential children are not means at all. Even those who remain agnostic about whether the human embryo is fully one of us should see the ways in which conducting such research would make us a different society: less humble toward that which we cannot fully understand, less willing to extend the boundaries of human respect ever outward, and more willing to transgress moral boundaries that we have, ourselves, so recently established, once it appears to be in our own interests to do so. We find it disquieting, even somewhat ignoble, to treat what are in fact seeds of the next generation as mere raw material for satisfying the needs of our own. Doing so would undermine the very prudence and humility to which defenders of limited embryo research often appeal: the idea that, while a human embryo may not be fully one of us, it is not humanly nothing and therefore should not be treated as a resource alone. But that is precisely what cloning-for-biomedical-research would do.

3. Opening the Door to Other Moral Hazards

This leads directly to our third concern—that the cloning of human embryos for research will open the door to additional (and to some of us, far greater) moral hazards. Human suffering from horrible diseases never comes to an end, and, likewise, our willingness to use embryonic life in the cause of research, once permitted, is also unlikely to find any natural stopping point. To set foot on this slope is to tempt ourselves to become people for whom the use of nascent human life as research material becomes routinized and everyday. That much is inherent in the very logic of what we would do in cloning-for-biomedical-research.

In addition, the reasons justifying production of cloned embryos for research can be predicted to expand. Today, the demand is for stem cells; tomorrow it may be for embryonic and fetal organs. The recent experiments with cloned cow embryos implanted in a cow's uterus[12] already suggest that there may be greater therapeutic potential using differentiated tissues (for example, kidney primordia) harvested from early fetuses than using undifferentiated stem cells taken from the very early embryo. Should this prove to be the case, pressure will increase to grow cloned human blastocysts to later stages—either in the uteruses of suitably prepared animal hosts or (eventually) using artificial placenta-like structures in the laboratory—in order to obtain the more useful tissues. One can even imagine without difficulty how a mother might be willing to receive into her womb as a temporary resident the embryonic clone of her desperately ill child, in order to harvest for that child life-saving organs or tissues. In such ways the coarsening of our moral sensibilities can be the fruit of understandable desires. Indeed, to refuse such further steps in the name of moral wisdom might come to seem increasingly sentimental, and, even if we were reluctant to give our approval, we might be hard-pressed to say why.

We should not be self-deceived about our ability to set limits on the exploitation of nascent life. What disturbs us today we quickly or eventually get used to; yesterday's repugnance gives way to tomorrow's endorsement. A society that already tolerates the destruction of fetuses in the second and third trimesters will hardly be horrified by embryo and fetus farming (including in animal wombs), if this should turn out to be helpful in the cure of dreaded diseases.

We realize, of course, that many proponents of cloning-for-biomedical-research will recommend regulations designed to prevent just such abuses (that is, the expansion of research to later-stage cloned embryos and fetuses). Refusing to erect a red light to stop research cloning, they will propose various yellow lights intended to assure ourselves that we are proceeding with caution, limits, or tears. Paradoxically, however, the effect might actually be to encourage us to continue proceeding with new (or more hazardous) avenues of research; for, believing that we are being cautious, we have a good conscience about what we do, and we are unable to imagine ourselves as people who could take a morally disastrous next step. We are neither wise enough nor good enough to live without clear limits.

Cloning-for-biomedical-research could require thousands of human eggs and would, as presently contemplated, give rise, as we have said, to a new industry of embryo manufacture. This industry would depend on eggs procured from women, themselves participants in the research, who would need to take drugs stimulating ovulation and to submit to the egg retrieval procedure. One might wonder whether their informed consent is sufficient to permit this in circumstances where, in the very nature of the case, the research is so preliminary that it cannot possibly provide effective therapies for patients. We might also worry lest women who are potential donors (because, for example, they have sought in vitro fertilization) might be vulnerable to pressure to participate in this research or financial inducements to do so. Even if such pressure does not rise to the level of coercion, we should acknowledge that there are inducements a just society would not offer and risks it would not ask potential research subjects—themselves vulnerable for a variety of reasons—to accept.

To get around the shortage of human eggs and the ethical dilemmas it could produce, scientists are exploring the possibility of substituting animal eggs in the initial cloning step of SCNT. Experiments creating animal-human hybrid-embryos, produced by inserting human DNA into enucleated rabbit oocytes, have already been conducted in China, with development up to the blastocyst stage.[13] Yet far from solving our ethical dilemma, the use of animal eggs raises new concerns about animal-human hybrids. We have no idea where these and later interspecies experiments might lead. Yet the creation of such chimeras, even in embryonic form, shows how ready we seem to be to blur further the boundary—biological and moral—between human being and animal.

Finally, if we accept even limited uses of cloning-for-biomedical-research, we significantly increase the likelihood of cloning-to-produce-children. The technique will gradually be perfected and the cloned embryos will become available, and those who would be interested in producing cloned children will find it much easier to do so. The only way to prevent this from happening would be to prohibit, by law, the implantation of cloned embryos for the purpose of producing children. To do so, however, the government would find itself in the unsavory position of designating a class of embryos that it would be a felony not to destroy. It would *require*, not just permit, the destruction of cloned embryos—which seems to us the very opposite of showing such cloned embryos "special respect."

4. Conclusion: What Prudence Requires

As history so often demonstrates, powers gained for one purpose are often used for other, less noble ones. We are about to harness powers over our own (human) nature to be used for our own well-intentioned purposes. But the knowledge that provides this power does not teach us how to use it. And given our fallibility, that should give us pause. We should consider, in making our moral judgment about cloning-for-biomedical-research, not simply the origin of these cells, but their possible uses (and misuses), as well as their place in the larger story of our increasing technological powers. We must keep in mind not simply where we took these cells from, but where they might take us, and what might be done with them.

In light of these moral and prudential dangers—namely, the crossing of the boundary from sexual to asexual reproduction; the possible misuse of our new genetic powers over embryonic life; the reduction of human embryos to nothing more than a resource and the coarsening of our moral sensibilities that would come with it; the prospect of a law that would mandate the destruction of nascent human life; and the prospect of other (greater) harms down the road, most notably the production of cloned children, research on later-stage fetuses, or genetic engineering of future generations—we must take pause and resist. In trying to discern where a wise and prudent boundary must be drawn—to protect those beings who are humanly inviolable, to prevent the dangers that most tempt us, and to protect the moral fabric of society—we hold that the boundary must be drawn by prohibiting the production and use of cloned embryos. To cross this boundary or to set it further down the road—that is, "with limits"—is to invite (and perhaps ensure) that some (or all) of the dehumanizing possibilities described above will come to pass.

C. What We Owe to the Suffering

The final question to be considered is what we owe to the suffering. Like our colleagues who endorse cloning-for-biomedical-research, we believe it would be less than human to turn a blind eye to those who suffer and need relief, or to stand silent in the face (especially) of suffering and premature death. In saying "no" to cloning-for-biomedical-research, we are not closing the door on medical progress—not in principle and not in practice. We are simply acknowledging that, for very strong moral reasons, progress must come by means that do not involve the production, use, and destruction of cloned embryos and that do not reduce nascent human life to a resource for our exploitation. This does mean, of course, that advances in basic research and progress in the cure of disease, though not halted, might be slowed (though, as described above, this is far from certain on scientific grounds). It is possible that some might suffer in the future because research proceeded more slowly. We cannot suppose that the moral life comes without cost. And honesty compels us not to offer guarantees where our human limits—and the unpredictable nature of the future—ensure that no such assurances are possible.

There may be occasions in life when the only means available for achieving a desired end is a means that it would be wrong to employ. This is especially true in circumstances such as those considered here; for to give our initial approval to cloning-for-biomedical-research is to set foot on a path whose deepest implications can scarcely be calculated. People sometimes imagine that human beings are responsible for all the harms they could prevent but do not; yet, this cannot be true. When we refuse to achieve a good outcome by doing what is wrong, and thereby perhaps accept some suffering that might have been avoided, we are not guilty of causing that suffering. To say otherwise would mean that sufficiently evil men could always hold us morally hostage. In order to obligate us to do an evil deed, they need only credibly threaten to do great harm unless we comply. Were we actually responsible for all the harm we might have prevented but did not, they would have us in their moral power. If our duty to prevent harm and suffering were always overriding, if it always held moral trump, we could not live nobly and justly.

We are not deaf to the voices of those who desperately want biomedical research to proceed. Indeed, we can feel the force of that desire ourselves, for all of us—and those we love most—are or could one day be patients desperate for a cure. But we are not only patients or potential patients. We are human beings and citizens, and we know that relief of suffering, though a great good, is not the greatest good. As highly as we value health and longer life, we know that life itself loses its value if we care only for *how long* we live, and not also for *how* we live.

Suppose, then, that we refrain from such research and that future sufferers say to us: "You might have helped us by approving cloning for research, but you declined to do so." What could we say to them? Something like the following: "Yes, perhaps so. But we could have done so only by destroying, in the present, the sort of world in which both we and you want to live—a world in which, as best we can, we respect human life and human individuals, the weak and the strong. To have done it would have meant stepping across boundaries that are essential to our humanity. And, although we very much want to leave to our children a world in which suffering can be more effectively relieved, that is not all we want to leave them. We want to bequeath to them a world that honors moral limits, a world in which the good of some human lives is not entirely subordinated to the good of others, a world in which we seek to respect, as best we can, the time each human being has and the place each fills."

This understanding of what commitment to our shared humanity requires is not alien to the efforts of scientific researchers to make progress in the cure of disease and relief of suffering. Theirs is, after all, a moral mission, which serves us all and which we all support. But if history teaches anything, it is the danger of assuming that, because our motives are praiseworthy and our hope is to heal, our actions cannot possibly violate or diminish human well-being. Indeed, we may be least likely to see the dangers when we are most confident of the goodness of our cause.

Scientists already accept important moral boundaries in research on human subjects, and they do not regard such boundaries as unwarranted restrictions on the freedom of scientific research. More generally, the scientific enterprise is a moral one not only because of the goals scientists seek but also because of the limits they honor. Indeed, it is precisely the acceptance of limits that stimulates creative advance, that forces scientists to conceive of new and morally acceptable ways of conducting research. Surely, therefore, before society takes a step that cannot be undone, it should ponder soberly the moral implications of accepting cloning, even for research.

To approve cloning-for-biomedical-research, to drink from that cup, is an inviting prospect indeed, but there is a spider in the cup. When we consider what we owe to the embryo, to our society, and to the suffering, we can see it more clearly and can, perhaps, acquire the wisdom and even the courage not to put this cup to our lips.

*   *   *

V. Conclusion

In this chapter, Council Members have presented as best we can the moral cases for and against cloning-for-biomedical-research, seen in the contexts of efforts to heal the sick; present and projected developments in reproductive, developmental, and genetic biotechnology; and the moral concerns for nascent life and the moral well-being of American society. Our different moral outlooks and judgments have been preserved and, we hope, clarified. We are now ready to move from ethics to public policy, in search of the best course of action regarding human cloning.

ENDNOTES

1 Osler, W. "Chauvinism in Medicine" *Aequanimitas, with Other Addresses to Medical Students, Nurses and Practitioners of Medicine* Philadelphia: Blakiston, 1943, p. 267.

2 For more information about the scientific and medical case for cloning-for-biomedical-research, see the following two reports: (1) National Research Council/Institute of Medicine (NRC/IOM), *Stem Cells and the Future of Regenerative Medicine,* Washington DC, National Academy Press, 2001. (2) National Academy of Sciences (NAS), *Scientific and Medical Aspects of Human Reproductive Cloning,* Washington, DC, National Academy Press, 2002.

3 Reyes, M., et al. "Origin of endothelial progenitors in human postnatal bone marrow" *Journal of Clinical Investigation,* 109: 337-346, 2002.

4 Jiang, Y. et al. "Pluripotency of mesenchymal stem cells derived from adult marrow" *Nature,* 418: 41-49, 2002.

5 Rideout III, W.M. et al. "Correction of a genetic defect by nuclear transplantation and combined cell and gene therapy" *Cell,* 109: 17-27, 2002.

6 Wilson, J.Q. "On Abortion" *Commentary,* 97(1): 21ff, 1994.

7 Lanza, R.P., et al. "Generation of histocompatible tissues using nuclear transplantation" *Nature Biotechnology,* 20: 689-696, 2002.

8 Brian Appleyard calls attention to this passage in his book, *Brave New Worlds: Staying Human in the Genetic Future* (New York: Viking, 1998).

9 Cited in Kass, L. "The Meaning of Life—in the Laboratory" *The Public Interest*, No. 146, pp. 45-46, Winter 2002.

10 Jonas, H. "Philosophical Reflections on Experimenting With Human Subjects" in *Readings on Ethical and Social Issues in Biomedicine,* ed. Richard W. Wertz (Prentice-Hall, 1973), p. 32.

11 National Bioethics Advisory Commission, *Ethical Issues in Human Stem Cell Research,* volume I, p. 53. Bethesda, MD: Government Printing Office, 1999.

12 See endnote 7, above.

13 Leggett, K., and A. Regalado. "China Stem Cell Research Surges as Western Nations Ponder Ethics" *Wall Street Journal,* March 6, 2002, p. A1.

Chapter Seven

Public Policy Options

The connection between moral assessment and public policy, here as elsewhere, is hardly straightforward. The relation of morality to law is notoriously complex, especially in free societies such as our own in which citizens may live their lives according to their own moral views. At the same time, however, practices deemed seriously wrong and harmful are outlawed, from incest and sexual abuse to slavery and racial discrimination. In addition, law functions not only to encourage or discourage conduct but also as a moral teacher. It expresses the social norms of the community, whether by fostering public education and medical research or by discouraging dishonest business practices and teenage pregnancy. Whether and how the law should address any given morally charged topic is often a debatable matter, requiring careful study and prudent judgment. Not everything that is morally defensible should be encouraged by public policy; not everything that is morally troubling should be legally proscribed.

These general remarks apply also to the case at hand. The moral assessments of the previous two chapters do not carry self-evident policy recommendations. Even a thoroughly developed moral position on either or both of the uses of human cloning still leaves open the question of what public policy would be appropriate, prudent, and effective. One can be morally opposed to cloning-to-produce-children, yet also oppose making it illegal, say, because of hesitation to increase the police power of the state in matters of reproduction. Or one can have no personal moral objection to cloning-for-biomedical-research, but still find practical reasons to favor a moratorium on such activity, say, because one wants to develop regulatory institutions before allowing the research to proceed. Moral principle and judgment, though necessary, are not sufficient for deliberating about what to do about human cloning. Prudence is also required.

In this chapter, we consider a broad range of public policy options. We assess and compare these options in the hope of seeing our way clear, in the eighth and final chapter of this report, to offer recommendations that comport, not only with our ethical judgments, but also with our sense as citizens of what is prudent, practical, and appropriate for this country at this time.

The policy debate about human cloning is a particularly vivid example of the tension between competing public goods, between the goods served by biomedical science and technology and other moral and social goods important to community life. The desire to ban human cloning, whether for producing children or for biomedical research, arises primarily from moral and social objections made in the name of human dignity, individuality, and respect for life. The opposition to a comprehensive ban on human cloning arises primarily from a belief that cloning research may lead to new remedies for human diseases and disabilities, backed also by appeals to the principle of freedom for scientific inquiry and technological innovation. Assumptions about the relative merits of these competing goods, as well as about the broader relation between science and society, lie just beneath the surface of this debate. Wittingly or not, these assumptions inform how people think about the various policy options proposed for dealing with human cloning. A brief examination of the more general question of the relation between science and society might clarify the principles that should guide our approach to a national policy on human cloning.

I. Science and Society

Since its birth in the seventeenth century, modern science—and especially modern medicine—has been guided by a desire to improve and elevate the human condition. Unlike ancient science, which sought speculative knowledge of *what things are* purely as an end in itself satisfying to the knower, modern science from the start sought effective knowledge of *how things work*, in the service of what Francis Bacon called "the conquest of nature for the relief of man's estate." Since then, scientists have been increasingly motivated not only by a deep desire *to know*, but also by a desire *to do*: that is, to provide resources, know-how, and relief in humanity's pursuit of health, happiness, and comfort. Biomedical scientists especially have pursued a dual goal: to increase our knowledge and understanding of living nature and to help the sick and the suffering.

In exchange for the promise of great human benefits, the practice of science entered into an unprecedented relation to the larger society. Scientists gradually acquired a privileged standing in modern societies, first with protections against persecution and censorship, later with public recognition and financial support. But it deserves to be noted that, insofar as the public respect for science rests on its moral intention and its ability to deliver the goods that society wants, scientists tacitly subject themselves to public scrutiny and moral judgment of their work, both as to ends and to means. The tacit social contract between scientists and society—freedom and support for scientists, benefits for all humanity—is double-sided: on the one hand, the opportunity for scientists to be public benefactors and recognized as such; on the other hand, the need, in cases where values conflict, for scientists to defend what they do in terms of the community's judgments about the relation of scientific activity to other moral and social goods.

As we have noted in the previous chapters, in the twentieth century, biomedical science made tremendous advances, resulting in both greater knowledge of how the human body works and greater ability to affect its workings. The results have been so dramatic, and so beneficial, that in the United States today virtually no one questions the benefits of the modern scientific endeavor, especially in medicine. This consensus about benefits has expressed itself as consistently strong public support for public funding of basic research, as well as strong support for the freedom of scientists to set their own research agendas, limited only by their curiosity, their imaginations, and our commonly agreed-upon moral and ethical norms. The tacit "contract" or relationship between science and society recognizes and celebrates the great benefits of freedom for all involved.

But for all these great benefits and good purposes, there are also times when the activities of scientists or the products of scientific work can imperil society and its members. For one thing, the work of scientific research is by its nature experimental. Scientific inquiry involves action, not only observation or theory. For this reason, *freedom of inquiry* does not adequately describe the freedom that scientific work requires and is generally granted. It may be more accurate to say that scientists desire and often receive great *freedom of action*. Yet because scientists learn by doing, some of what scientists do can be dangerous or inappropriate. And because some of their actions may infringe on the rights, security, or dignity of individuals, or on the principles and interests of society as a whole, scientific freedom of action cannot be absolute.

In addition, many of the technological products of scientific research can be used to do harm as well as good. Just as society has moved in the past to restrict access to dangerous nuclear and biological agents, as well as to restrict public access to information about these things, so too will society be confronted with moral challenges by the new biomedical technologies. Technologies that disclose our genetic abnormalities or that alter the human genome, neurotropic drugs that can enhance (or destroy) memory or libido, computer implants in human brains—these and many other technological possibilities now on the horizon may raise profound moral and social challenges to privacy, freedom, equality, dignity, and human self-understanding. As citizens we may—indeed we must—decide whether and where to limit potentially harmful research or technology even as we continue to desire and uphold free intellectual inquiry and technological innovation.

American society has done this in the past. The various codes of conduct for human experimentation, discussed at several points in this report, demonstrate some of the ways in which the polity has established important moral boundaries that biomedical researchers must respect. In addition, rules and restrictions governing the pharmaceutical industry, the practice of medicine, the sale of organs for transplantation, the handling of biohazards, the development of biological weapons, and numerous other areas of scientific and technological work show that even given our desire for scientific advance and our belief in the inherent value of freedom, the pursuit of research and technology has not been allowed to trump all other concerns.

Thus we conclude that in the realm of genetics and reproduction, as in many others, boundaries and regulations may be needed: lines may need to be drawn that none may cross, guidelines may need to be established that all must follow. Because the wisdom needed to decide how scientific knowledge and technology should be used is not something that science can provide by itself, these boundaries and regulations must be set by the whole community, democratically, through its representative institutions, and not only by those who are experts in the scientific work involved. Our analysis in Chapters Five and Six of the serious moral and social questions raised by human cloning has persuaded us that human cloning in *both* its forms is an appropriate area for public policy.

II. Public Policy Options: General Considerations

A. The Scope of Policy

Having decided that human cloning is an activity fit for public policy decision, we still face many questions. Does it warrant legislative proscription, governmental regulation, professional oversight or self-regulation, or merely civil tort liability for bad results? And how broadly or narrowly should we delimit the domain in which human cloning is to be considered? Although the ethical analysis in this report has often concentrated on human cloning considered on its own, when considering public policy it is especially important to recall the larger contexts in which human cloning belongs. As we emphasized in Chapters One and Two, human cloning (in both its possible uses) would be but a special area of a larger domain of biotechnology, made possible by present and projected techniques of embryo research, assisted reproduction, genetic screening, and genetic engineering—all of which are coming to be grouped under the field of "reprogenetics." As we contemplate possible policy options regarding human cloning, it behooves us to consider what cloning's place within this broader context might mean for public policy.

Many other countries have in fact taken up cloning in this broader context. In Germany, for example, this broader approach has taken the form of a series of legal proscriptions and restrictions, centered on the Embryo Protection Act of 1990. The act treats all embryo research together and prohibits all interventions not undertaken for the well-being of the embryo (including the creation of embryos specifically for research). The German system also includes specific rules for IVF procedures, and in general treats all interventions involving the human embryo under one rubric. Human cloning, for whatever purposes, is legislatively prohibited.

In the United Kingdom, too, policy on these subjects takes as its organizing principle the human embryo itself, though the approach here is regulative rather than proscriptive. The British system is centered around a regulatory body—the Human Fertilization and Embryology Authority (HFEA), created in 1990—charged with monitoring and regulating essentially all of what has come to be called reprogenetics, including human cloning, both for producing children and for biomedical research. The HFEA regulates infertility treatment and clinical work; storage of gametes and embryos; and all embryo research, whether publicly or privately funded. It licenses these various activities, monitors compliance, sets standards of practice, establishes limits and requirements on the use of embryos for various purposes, and maintains a detailed information registry about both assisted reproduction and embryo research. Human cloning is treated within this broader regulatory scheme: cloning-to-produce-children is not permitted; cloning-for-biomedical-research is allowed, but only with cloned embryos no older than fourteen days.

Canada is completing the process of establishing a national system, combining elements of legal proscription and governmental regulation, to govern all technological activities used to help people have children as well as the use of embryos in research. Some activities would be permitted and regulated, others would be prohibited by law. The chosen point of departure is not the human embryo, but rather the goods of human health and dignity: to protect the health and safety of Canadians; to prevent commercial exploitation of reproduction; and to protect human individuality and diversity and the integrity of the human genome. A single broad regulatory body, the Assisted Human Reproduction Agency of Canada, would issue and renew licenses for assisted reproduction facilities, collect and analyze health information, set policies, and monitor compliance. Among the prohibited activities are all human cloning, whether to produce children or for biomedical research. Human embryos no longer needed for infertility may be used for stem cell research (with consent of the progenitors). But producing in vitro embryos for research purposes is prohibited, except for efforts to improve assisted reproduction procedures.[1]

Several other countries have approached this area of biotechnology with a similar broad outlook. The United States to date has not; indeed we lack any national monitoring, oversight, or regulatory system in this area. It may therefore be appropriate, in connection with thinking about specific policies for human cloning in the United States, to initiate discussions of a national policy for these related arenas. Doing so might allow us to regard the question of embryo research in its full scope, and to consider it together with the closely related issues that arise when the techniques of assisted reproduction come together with those of genetic diagnosis and potential genetic engineering. In putting forward its recommendations in the next chapter, the Council will take into account this broader context of related biotechnologies.

Yet, much as it would be desirable to consider public policy regarding human cloning in its larger context, it is for us also necessary to consider it on its own. Owing to the immediate concern over the prospect of cloning-to-produce-children, legislative proposals and public debate have largely treated the subject of human cloning in isolation—though for reasons we have noted, it has overlapped with the controversy about embryonic stem cell research. Accordingly, the policy options presented below are drawn for the most part from the ongoing public and legislative debate about human cloning, and therefore direct themselves to legislative alternatives regarding cloning in particular.

B. A Legislative Complication

There is a complication that bedevils prospects for legislation regarding human cloning. Given that human cloning may be used for two very different purposes—to produce children and for biomedical research—one might think that these two different uses could be treated independently, just as we have done (for the most part) in the ethical analyses in Chapters Five and Six. The ethical issues of cloning-to-produce-children and cloning-for-biomedical-research differ considerably, and, as our own discussions have indicated, one's moral assessment of the second can be independent of one's moral assessment of the first. Some people who oppose cloning-to-produce-children may favor cloning-for-biomedical-research; some people who oppose producing embryos solely for research may object less forcefully to cloning-to-produce-children (should it ever become safe to attempt it). And people who oppose both uses may differ as to which they think is the worse. Given these variations, it would seem sensible to disaggregate the two forms of cloning and develop independent public policies for each.

But this is easier said than done. The reason is simple: both forms begin in the same way with the act of cloning (by somatic cell nuclear transfer [SCNT]) that produces a cloned human embryo. It is therefore difficult—perhaps impossible—to craft a public policy regarding one use of cloned human embryos that does not, at least tacitly but usually explicitly, also affect the other. A thoroughgoing attempt to prevent cloning-to-produce-children by banning the first step would also prevent cloning-for-biomedical-research. An attempt to promote cloning-for-biomedical-research might well have consequences for cloning-to-produce-children (for example, by improving the technique or by increasing the likelihood of attempts to initiate a pregnancy). An attempt to prevent cloning-to-produce-children at the step of transfer of a cloned embryo to initiate a pregnancy would tacitly approve the initial creation of cloned embryos for other purposes. Moreover, by imposing penalties on implantation while sanctioning creation, a policy that banned only transfer to a uterus would in effect require, by law, that cloned human embryos be destroyed.

Even if one thinks only of the task of statutory drafting, the difficulty persists. For if one wants to make a particular action illegal, one must specify precisely the act to be proscribed. It turns out to be very difficult to specify precisely and unambiguously the forbidden act of human cloning without touching both uses at once. "It shall be unlawful to attempt to clone a human being" is simple enough to say, but vexing to specify. The meaning of the term "human being" is contested: does it mean only a child or adult, or is an embryo too a human being, albeit in its primordial stage? The definition of "to clone" must specify either the initial act of somatic cell nuclear transfer or the birth of a cloned child. "*Attempting* to clone" will mean either somatic cell nuclear transfer itself or the transfer of the resulting cloned embryo to a woman's uterus.

There is, of course, one possible policy approach that could disentangle the two uses of human cloning, but it would require dealing with cloning-for-biomedical-research in a different context. Since cloning-for-biomedical-research is one form of embryo research—another is research that uses embryos produced by IVF—one could have a broad policy on *all* embryo research, which would then necessarily apply to research with *cloned* embryos. Several states have separate laws that cover research on all human embryos, cloned or not. In these cases, a law to deal with the special practice of cloning-to-produce-children could then be added without difficulty. And, as we have indicated, in the United Kingdom and several other countries, there is a broad regulatory system for handling all activities involving human embryos—both for research and for initiating pregnancies—into which further regulations regarding *cloned* embryos may easily be fit. But the legislative debates in Congress, both in 1998 and in 2001-2002, have not squarely addressed independent treatment of embryo research in general and cloning-for-biomedical-research in particular. That fact shapes our examination of specific public policy options.

III. Public Policy Options: Specific Alternatives

What *sort* of policy regarding human cloning would be most appropriate in this country at this time? In approaching the various alternatives, we operate on the following premises.

First, given the seriousness of the subject, we favor a policy that makes an explicit and considered decision about whether to proceed. Should our society come to have *no* rules or guidelines regarding human cloning, it should do so deliberately, not by default.

Second, we need to decide *whose* decision and responsibility this should be. And while we may differ among ourselves on the answer to this question, we agree that whichever persons, institutions, or agencies of government have authority for the decision and any subsequent oversight, the responsible parties should be answerable to and held accountable by the people and their representatives. This is not an arena where secrecy or lack of accountability should be tolerated.

Third, whether one opts for permission with or without regulation or for legislative proscription, permanent or temporary, we believe that the following two balancing principles should be followed: (1) Because of the gravity of the issues at stake, whoever bears the power of decision needs to be persuaded that we should *now* proceed with human cloning, in either or both of its forms. (2) At the same time, we should not stand in the way of proceeding simply out of some vague fear of possible future harms of unknown magnitude; we should interfere only if the harms are deemed serious, important to the common good, and likely to occur.

A. Federal or State Jurisdiction?

We begin, as we should in America, by examining human cloning in the context of our constitutional system and, in particular, of our special form of federalism. In short, we must consider which level of government has jurisdiction. Human cloning is not obviously a federal concern, nor is it plainly outside the jurisdiction of the states; thus it might be presumed to be a matter for regulation by the states alone. Certainly a number of states have moved to legislate in this area. As of this writing, twenty-two state legislatures have considered bills on cloning, and six of them have passed laws on the subject. Of these, five directly or indirectly prohibit both forms of human cloning, while one prohibits only cloning-to-produce-children.* It is possible to argue that human cloning is one of those many issues, essentially local in nature, that call more or less exclusively for the exercise of local self-government, which in the American system means primarily government by the states. And yet, a number of factors point to the need to consider a federal policy as well.

For one thing, as we hope the foregoing chapters have made clear, human cloning-to-produce-children has nationwide implications, with potentially profound effects on individuals, families, and all of society. This view is reflected in the efforts in

---

* As of June 2002, three states (Iowa, Michigan, and Virginia) ban both cloning-to-produce-children and cloning-for-biomedical-research. Two states (Louisiana and Rhode Island) ban cloning-to-produce-children, but also have embryo-research laws that appear to prohibit cloning-for-biomedical-research. One state (California) has banned cloning-to-produce-children until December 31, 2002, but has no embryo-research law and thus effectively permits cloning-for-biomedical-research.

Congress to legislate on the subject, first in 1998 and again in 2001 and 2002. President Clinton made clear, in his executive order on human cloning,[2] that he regards it as a federal issue; and President Bush has done likewise in several public statements.[3]

For another thing, the federal government plays an extensive role in funding and regulating scientific research. Insofar as there has been a role for government in the oversight of scientific work in America, it has generally been filled by the federal government, for reasons of scale and efficacy and also to some extent of historical accident. So long as this remains the case, questions relating to the funding and regulation of human cloning will, in practice, be addressed mostly or even solely at the federal level.

Moreover, it can be assumed that, if they remain legally permissible, both forms of human cloning would tend to enter into interstate commerce, thus bringing them within the purview of Congress, at least as far as its power to regulate interstate commerce allows.

Historically, when several or most of the states have proscribed some activity they regard as injurious to public health, safety, or morals (such as prostitution or the use of narcotic drugs), the federal government has tended to enact laws supportive of the states', or most of the states', moral proscriptions, either by restricting interstate commerce (as in the Mann Act relating to prostitution) or even by directly prohibiting the activity itself (as in the Federal Controlled Substances Act). Since the states have begun to act on human cloning, it has become valid therefore to ask whether federal legislation is also needed.

Finally, human cloning has become a subject of international law. A number of nations have moved to prohibit one or both forms of human cloning, and the United Nations is currently debating whether to promulgate an international convention to ban cloning-to-produce-children. Since only the federal government can make treaties or conduct foreign policy for the whole nation, it seems likely that at some point the United—and not merely the separate—States will be under pressure to legislate on this subject.

For some or all of these reasons, we think it reasonable to conclude that human cloning, of either variety, is a fit subject for debate and action at the federal level.[*]

B. Seven Basic Policy Options

With respect to each form of human cloning, cloning-to-produce-children and cloning-for-biomedical-research, there are two basic alternatives: permit or prohibit. For each of these alternatives, there are again two further possibilities: permit with or without regulation; prohibit indefinitely ("ban") or for a limited time ("moratorium"). (The alternative "permit with regulation" might or might not make permission contingent upon getting the regulatory system *in place beforehand*.) Among the numerous permutations and possibilities, we now take up seven basic policy options that have been publicly discussed and that appear to us worthy of consideration:

- *Policy Option 1:* Professional self-regulation with no legislative action ("self-regulation").

- *Policy Option 2:* A ban on cloning-to-produce-children, with neither endorsement nor restriction of cloning-for-biomedical-research ("ban plus silence").

---

[*] We prescind from trying to determine at length whether federal legislation limiting human cloning would infringe on what some believe is a fundamental constitutional right to attempt to procreate. Nor will we try to offer our own legal opinion about whether the Food and Drug Administration has existing authority that would enable it to regulate either or both forms of human cloning. These questions we are content to leave to others. Instead we proceed here on the assumption that, whatever the precise state of the law, Congress may (and we would argue, should) take the lead in determining federal cloning policy.

- *Policy Option 3:* A ban on cloning-to-produce-children, with regulation of the use of cloned embryos for biomedical research ("ban plus regulation").

- *Policy Option 4:* Governmental regulation, perhaps by a new federal agency, with no legislative prohibitions ("regulation of both").

- *Policy Option 5:* A ban on all human cloning, whether to produce children or for biomedical research ("ban on both").

- *Policy Option 6:* A ban on cloning-to-produce-children, with a moratorium, or temporary ban, on cloning-for-biomedical-research ("ban plus moratorium").

- *Policy Option 7:* A moratorium, or temporary ban, on all human cloning, whether to produce children or for biomedical research ("moratorium on both").

In considering each of these options, we bear in mind four basic questions: (1) How would the policy be enforced and by whom? (2) On what moral opinions, and on what views of the role of government, is it based? (3) What are the arguments in favor? (4) What are the possible objections? To avoid needless repetition, where two options are very similar we refrain from repeating the same arguments at great length, and instead focus on the major new points worthy of note.

*   *   *

<u>*Policy Option 1*</u>: *Professional self-regulation with no legislative action ("self-regulation").*

This option would enact no new legal restraints on human cloning, and rely instead on self-regulation and private decision making. Passing no law on the subject would maintain the legal status quo; it would leave in place the existing moratorium on federal funding for either form of human cloning, while also leaving private parties free to use private funds to conduct either form of human cloning, as they see fit, consistent with state law.

This approach would let physicians and patients decide privately whether to engage in cloning-to-produce-children[*] It would rely upon the people actually engaged in cloning-for-biomedical-research to establish a mechanism for self-regulation and to prevent abuses. And it could utilize tort liability to deter tragedies and mishaps, by holding people legally responsible for harms inflicted upon a cloned child or his or her mother.

This approach assumes that neither form of human cloning poses moral or practical dangers sufficient to require public action. It assumes that the harms of cloning-to-produce-children are not so grave as to merit a legal restriction, and it sees no harm, or at least negligible harm, in cloning-for-biomedical-research. It also assumes that government's role in regulating scientific research and reproductive medicine should be minimal; that federal legislation may cause more harms than it prevents; that self-regulation provides sufficient safeguards against the worst abuses of cloning practices; that the subject is so complex that the people best qualified to regulate it are the experts in the field themselves; or that any more restrictive policy is unlikely to succeed and likely to drive scientific talent overseas to more permissive jurisdictions.

---

[*] The Food and Drug Administration (FDA) has stated that attempts to clone humans would come under its jurisdiction. But this assertion of regulatory authority has never been tested, and might well be disputed if it were invoked in practice. The FDA has never attempted to regulate the human uses of IVF embryos.

This hands-off approach would seem to ignore the widespread public and congressional support for a ban on cloning-to-produce-children, as evidenced in the July 31, 2001, vote in the House of Representatives, where nearly every member voted for some kind of federal ban on at least one form of human cloning. Of this option, it may be asked: Is cloning-to-produce-children so morally unproblematic that we could safely leave people free to try it? Would tort liability really be sufficient to deter abuses? And can we afford a laissez-faire policy on what is surely only the first of a series of powerful new genetic technologies? For those who answer "no" to any of these questions, it will be necessary to seek another option.

Policy Option 2: A ban on cloning-to-produce-children, with neither endorsement nor restriction of cloning-for-biomedical-research ("ban plus silence").

A second option would be to prohibit cloning-to-produce-children but remain silent on cloning-for-biomedical-research. Such a policy would prohibit the implantation rather than the creation of cloned human embryos. By remaining silent on the question of creating cloned human embryos, this approach would not establish an oversight mechanism or other means of keeping track of cloned embryos or otherwise preventing implantation before the act itself is undertaken. It would therefore probably not require a new enforcement agency; enforcement of the ban would presumably fall to the Department of Justice.

This approach assumes that cloning-to-produce-children is sufficiently unacceptable as to merit legal prohibition, but minimizes or sets aside the disputed question of cloning-for-biomedical-research. It seeks to balance the responsibility for establishing public control over potential misuses of technology with public tolerance for competing worldviews and interests. It permits potentially valuable medical and scientific research to go forward. It preserves the current federal embryo-research policy, which (1) permits all embryo research to proceed unimpeded with private funds, (2) permits research on certain embryonic stem cell lines to proceed under federal guidance with public funds, and (3) leaves open, for continued debate, the question of whether there should be public funding for embryo and embryonic stem cell research.

Against this option, it can be argued that it is not possible for the government to be neutral on the question of cloning-for-biomedical-research. It is difficult, if not impossible, to write a statute banning the act of implanting cloned embryos without tacitly sanctioning the creation of the cloned embryos in the first place. Thus, a ban on cloning-to-produce-children not accompanied by a prohibition on cloning-for-biomedical-research would put the government in the position of allowing the creation of a class of (cloned) human embryos and then effectively mandating their destruction (or at least their perpetual preservation in cold storage), a class of (cloned) human embryos that it would be a felony to try to keep alive to birth. Also such a partial ban could arguably make cloning-to-produce-children more likely to occur. After all, without a regulatory system in place to keep track of and govern the use of cloned human embryos, the ban on implantation would be difficult to monitor and enforce. The commercial production of embryos for research would be protected by industrial secrecy. The transfer of cloned embryos to begin a pregnancy would be virtually undetectable and protected by doctor-patient confidentiality. Those charged with monitoring and enforcing the ban on cloning-to-produce-children would not know who is doing what with cloned human embryos. Moreover, actually enforcing the ban in the event of a violation would be nearly impossible. Once a clonal pregnancy has begun, there would be no real remedy except a forced abortion, an untenable option.

Policy Option 3: *A ban on cloning-to-produce-children, with regulation of the use of cloned embryos for biomedical research ("ban plus regulation").*

This option would be similar to Option 2 ("ban plus silence"), but in place of silence would require the establishment of a system of oversight and regulation of cloning-for-biomedical-research. These functions would be carried out by a regulatory agency (new or existing) authorized to do some or all of the following things:

1. Establish what may and may not be done with cloned human embryos once they are created, including a prohibition on implantation of cloned human embryos into human, animal, or artificial wombs.

2. License and conduct prior review of all research involving cloned embryos.

3. Establish guidelines for the protection of all human subjects participating in the research, including donors of eggs and nuclei.

4. Register and track each individual cloned human embryo.

5. Establish the number of days beyond which a cloned human embryo may not be grown in vitro, and enforce this requirement.

6. Monitor and regulate financial transactions regarding cloned embryos and human oocytes used in cloning-for-biomedical-research.

7. Monitor corporate, academic, and industrial cloning-for-biomedical-research, check for compliance, and enforce sanctions against violations of regulations.

To be effective, such a regulatory structure would have to be applied to both federally funded and privately funded research. Its first purpose would be to facilitate the ban on cloning-to-produce-children, by keeping close track of all research using cloned human embryos. Its second aim would be to enforce certain general standards for the handling and use of cloned human embryos, to ensure that they are not created for frivolous purposes, used irresponsibly, or treated in ways that go beyond what American society deems morally acceptable.

This option assumes that neutrality on the question of cloning-for-biomedical-research is neither possible nor desirable. Instead, it assumes that a system is needed to regulate and limit the use of cloned embryos—both in the interest of preventing cloning-to-produce-children, and in the interest of establishing a clear ethical framework for undertaking cloning-for-biomedical-research and allowing that research to flourish. At the same time, such a system would establish clear rules and limits to prevent abuses—for example, experimentation on later-stage embryos and fetuses or attempts to produce cloned children.

This new task could be assigned to an existing regulatory agency (or combination of agencies), such as the Food and Drug Administration or the National Institutes of Health, or, alternatively, it could be carried out by a new regulatory agency devised specifically for the purpose.

Establishment of a regulatory structure may be aided by the study of models in other countries, such as the United Kingdom's Human Fertilization and Embryology Authority (HFEA) or the Assisted Human Reproduction Agency being brought into existence in Canada—taking into account, of course, the important differences between their political, economic, and health-care systems and our own.

Regulation, for these proponents, would limit the uses of cloned embryos to especially promising and worthy biomedical research and would set boundaries beyond which such embryos may not be grown or exploited. For some proponents of this option, such oversight and regulation would be aimed primarily at preventing the use of cloned embryos to produce children. For others, regulation is called for to ensure that cloned human embryos be treated not simply as a natural resource but with appropriate measures of respect owed them as *human* embryos.

Against this option can be raised some of the same objections that were raised against Option 2 ("ban plus silence"), namely, that it puts the government in the new position of requiring the destruction of nascent human life, and that it could, by allowing the production of cloned human embryos, make cloning-to-produce-children more likely. It might also be argued against this option that setting up a workable regulatory structure is either impossible or impossible to do very quickly. After all, the IVF and assisted-reproduction industry is today largely unregulated in any way that could be called coordinated, comprehensive, or systematic. The federal government has no experience in regulating or keeping track of the number and fate of embryos produced in IVF clinics.* And the biotechnology industry has shown little enthusiasm for outside regulation. Establishing an effective regulatory regime could take several years of trial and error, during which time cloned embryos might be mishandled or implanted in an effort to produce children. There are also the dangers that regulatory bodies often prove ineffective and unaccountable and that they are vulnerable to capture by special interests that have a large stake, economic or other, in their regulatory decisions but little incentive to respect the permanent and aggregate interests of the nation. Establishing the regulatory body overseeing human cloning-for-biomedical-research within the National Institutes of Health, for example, would not be reassuring to those who worry that the fate of the embryo will always be subordinated to the imperative for research. In this view, regulation is not enough.

Policy Option 4: _Governmental regulation, perhaps by a new federal agency, with no legislative prohibitions ("regulation of both")._

This option is similar to the regulatory half of Option 3 ("ban plus regulation"), but the regulatory agency would have authority to set policy and guidelines also regarding cloning-to-produce-children. In addition to the functions listed in the description of

---

* The FDA has never attempted to regulate the practice of IVF, intracytoplasmic sperm injection, preimplantation genetic diagnosis, or embryo research conducted with IVF-produced embryos.

Option 3, the regulatory body would determine if and when human cloning techniques were sufficiently safe to warrant attempts to produce children by human cloning. The entity might also function as a licensing agency, setting down clear guidelines delineating acceptable and unacceptable purposes for such a practice (for example, it might choose to permit cloning to "replace" a deceased child but not to "replicate" a famous athlete).

The major argument for this option is flexibility: as the science and technology of human cloning proceeds in nonhuman animals, and as the public's views develop in response to new information and new debates, the nation will not be locked into a legislatively defined position that might later appear to have been misguided. Either a congressional ban or the refusal to enact a ban may prove to be a decision that will later look undesirable and yet difficult to undo.

Against this option are many of the same objections raised against the regulatory part of Option 3. Also, it may be argued that, given our society's strong moral opposition to cloning-to-produce-children, any decision to permit such a practice, even in exceptional cases, should not be left to a regulatory body; it should rather require a decision by people directly accountable to the voters. This option fails that test.

Policy Option 5: *A ban on all human cloning, whether to produce children or for biomedical research ("ban on both").*

This option would ban the initial act of human cloning—the production of cloned human embryos—regardless of the intended purpose. It would thus prohibit both forms of human cloning.

Specifically, this approach would proscribe the act of producing cloned human embryos by means of SCNT. Although enforcing the ban would be the responsibility of law enforcement agencies—as would enforcing a ban on cloning-to-produce-children—the "policing of laboratories" would hardly be necessary. Financial and criminal penalties, along with the inability to publish, patent, or profit from (the now illegal) work involving cloned human embryos, would by themselves eliminate nearly all incentive to clone. The ban would deter by subjecting to prosecution and social stigma any researchers or institutions whose efforts to create cloned human embryos came to public attention.

As we have seen in previous chapters, some proponents of this option argue that the creation, use, and ultimate destruction of cloned human embryos solely for research is morally unacceptable, either in itself or because of its moral consequences. Others hold that a ban only on the transferring of cloned embryos to a woman's uterus, even with additional regulations, would fail to prevent the cloning of a child, and that human cloning must be comprehensively stopped before it starts. Also, any regulatory arrangements that allowed cloning-for-biomedical-research within *legally* established limits would put the federal government in the novel and morally troubling position of mandating the destruction of nascent life.

In favor of this approach it can be argued that a "ban on both" would steer scientists toward less morally troubling (and, in the view of some, more medically promising) forms of biomedical research. Indeed, some argue that pursuing cloning-for-biomedical-research might actually hurt those patients whom it claims to help, by diverting valuable resources away from more promising areas of research or more urgent health-care needs. By taking this option, some proponents argue, America would send a strong signal of moral leadership to the rest of the world, where the human cloning question is also currently being debated.

Against this option it is frequently and vigorously argued that prohibiting cloning-for-biomedical-research would cut off a promising avenue of medical research. It is also argued that forbidding such research here may simply drive American talent overseas and thus diminish American scientific preeminence and economic strength.

<u>*Policy Option 6*</u>: *A ban on cloning-to-produce-children, with a moratorium, or temporary ban, on cloning-for-biomedical-research ("ban plus moratorium").*

This option would impose a permanent legal prohibition on cloning-to-produce-children, by banning the creation and subsequent transfer of cloned embryos into a woman's uterus. At the same time, it would also prohibit the creation of cloned human embryos for any reason, but would require a mandatory review of that latter prohibition after a certain period of time (for example, five years). This option would lock in a permanent ban on the activity virtually everyone opposes (cloning-to-produce-children), while calling for continued and enlarged debate on a question about which people currently differ (cloning-for-biomedical-research).

The main benefits of a moratorium on cloning-for-biomedical-research are that it would (1) allow time for research in related fields to proceed and perhaps clarify the potentially unique benefits of cloning-for-biomedical-research or discover superior alternatives that would make cloning-for-biomedical-research unnecessary; (2) allow time for a regulatory structure—whether narrow or broad in scope—to be developed, if deemed desirable; and (3) allow time for further debate and deliberation about the moral questions, to determine if the prohibition on cloning-for-biomedical-research should be renewed, made permanent, or abandoned after the moratorium expires. Rightly understood, a moratorium should not be seen as an attempt to stall, but as an opportunity to figure out the wisest way to proceed. And for those interested in exploring and establishing regulatory arrangements, a moratorium, as a *de jure* halt, would provide prospective researchers with an incentive (otherwise lacking) to recommend moral and legal guidelines before the moratorium would expire and be up for possible renewal.

This option separates cloning-to-produce-children from cloning-for-biomedical-research. It therefore would enable policymakers to take up the question of cloning-for-biomedical-research in the larger context of the embryo-research question, rather than in the narrower context of human cloning.

This option captures much of the current public debate, in which there is general agreement on the need to prohibit cloning for producing children, but a great deal of uncertainty over the proper approach to cloning-for-biomedical-research.

The arguments against this option are the same as those leveled against Option 5 ("ban on both"), namely, that prohibiting cloning-for-biomedical-research, even for a limited time, would cut off a promising avenue of medical research and simply drive American talent overseas. Others may object that the two uses of human cloning might hereafter be delinked, a prospect that troubles some for both practical and moral reasons (laid out in the discussion of the next option).

Policy Option 7: A moratorium, or temporary ban, on all human cloning, whether to produce children or for biomedical research ("moratorium on both").

The final option is a temporary form of Option 5 ("ban on both"), with a mandatory review of the policy after a certain period of time (for example, five years).

The main benefits of this option are the same as those listed above for Option 6 ("ban plus moratorium"). But this option has what some consider the additional virtue of keeping the two uses of cloning linked in the policy arena. This has, they say, two major benefits.

First, on *practical* grounds, the policy on cloning-for-biomedical-research will bear heavily on the feasibility and efficacy of any ban on cloning-to-produce-children, and therefore there is an advantage in ensuring that the two are considered together. Because the availability of cloned embryos would make enforcement of the ban on cloning-to-produce-children more complicated and demanding, a ban on cloning-to-produce-children should never be de-coupled from an identical ban on cloning-for-biomedical-research.

Second, on *moral* grounds, some argue that permitting the creation of cloned human embryos for research crosses an important line, and that one use of cloned embryos should not be separated fully from the other in public consideration. They hold that human cloning is a single thing, and therefore should be taken up whole. They are concerned that, at the end of the moratorium outlined in Option 6, the situation would be transformed into Option 2 ("ban plus silence") or Option 3 ("ban plus regulation"), with all the deficiencies that they think these permissive options would hold. For this reason, these opponents argue, it is more appropriate for both forms to be considered together at the end of the moratorium period, even if the eventual resulting policy does not treat them equally.

Once again, the arguments against this option are the same as those leveled against Option 5 ("ban on both") or Option 6 ("ban plus moratorium")—that it would cut off, at least temporarily, a promising avenue of medical research and drive American talent overseas. In addition, some may object that linking the two uses of cloning misrepresents the state of the public discussion on the subject and places cloning-for-biomedical-research in the wrong context—causing it to be considered always as a form of cloning, rather than as a form of embryo research.

Finally, some do not want to forgo the present opportunity to enact a *permanent* ban on cloning-to-produce-children; failure to do so now, they argue, would seem to imply that cloning-to-produce-children may one day be perfectly acceptable.

*   *   *

Having sketched out what we consider to be the most plausible options, we now proceed to offer our own policy recommendations and our reasons for them.

ENDNOTES

[1] Presentation made by Dr. Patricia Baird, chair, Royal Commission on New Reproductive Technologies, at the June 2002 meeting of the President's Council. Transcript available at the Council's web site, www.bioethics.gov.

[2] Clinton, W.J., "Memorandum on the Prohibition on Federal Funding for Cloning of Human Beings, March 4, 1997" In *Weekly Compilation of Presidential Documents* (Volume 33, Number 10), p. 281. Washington, DC: Government Printing Office, 1997.

[3] Bush, G.W., "Remarks on Human Cloning Legislation, April 10, 2002" In *Weekly Compilation of Presidential Documents* (Volume 38, Number 15), pp. 608-610. Washington, DC: Government Printing Office, 2002.

Chapter Eight

Policy Recommendations

The Council's formation of its policy recommendations is shaped by the following considerations:

First, our recognition of both the scientific and technological and the human and ethical contexts of human cloning, considered in Chapters One through Four.

Second, our awareness that human cloning is but a small part of a large and growing field of biomedical science and technology based on the convergence of developmental biology and genetics; and our awareness that this field offers relief for human disease and suffering while impinging also upon human procreation and family life, regard for nascent human life, and the relations between science and society.

Third, our ethical assessments of cloning-to-produce-children and cloning-for-biomedical-re-search, as presented in Chapters Five and Six.

Fourth, our ethical and prudential assessment of the strengths and weaknesses, benefits and harms, of the various policy options, as presented in Chapter Seven, including a serious effort to judge—in the face of unavoidable ignorance about what the future may bring—what will likely be gained and what will likely be lost should we pursue one path rather than another.

Fifth, our assessment of recent congressional efforts to develop national legislation on human cloning, and the reasons for their failures to date.

Sixth, our respect for the strongly held moral views of those with whom we do not agree, both on the Council and in the larger society.

Seventh, our desire to seek a wise and prudent course of action that does justice to our deepest moral concerns while preserving our nation's thriving biomedical science and technology.

I. The Council's Points of Departure in Formulating Policy Recommendations

(a) The Council regards the country's public policy decision about human cloning as a matter of great moment. It is important not only for its effect on the prospects of human cloning but also for what it will say about our democratic society's ability to govern the course of technological innovation and use in the name of things we as a nation hold dear.

(b) The Council is unanimous in opposing cloning-to-produce-children. We hold that the likely harms and injustices to prospective cloned offspring and the women involved, as well as to their families and the broader society, are sufficiently great and sufficiently likely as to justify governmental action to prevent cloning-to-produce-children.

(c) Two general approaches have thus far been proposed by those seeking to prevent cloning-to-produce-children. The first would stop the process at the first step by banning the creation of any cloned embryos. The second would stop the process at the initiation of a pregnancy by banning the transfer of a cloned embryo into a woman's uterus (or other gestational environment). If the question of cloning-to-produce-children were considered in isolation, the first and stricter ban would be most prudent: if it were illegal to produce cloned embryos, they would be less likely to be created and hence less likely to be available for attempts at pregnancy. But such a comprehensive ban would preclude cloning-for-biomedical-research, research favored by most scientists and patient advocacy groups, but about which the public is deeply divided.

(d) Regarding the ethics of cloning-for-biomedical-research, the Council is of many minds. Among Members who *approve* the practice—all of whom strongly endorse the worthiness and importance of the research and its enormous potential for medical therapies—a few approve it unconditionally and with enthusiasm, but more approve it with moral concern. Among the latter are a few Members who, though approving it in principle, are reluctant at this time to approve it in practice, for one or more of the following prudential reasons: the current lack of sufficient scientific evidence to sustain claims of the *unique* value of *cloned* embryos for the desired researches; the absence of proper regulatory institutions and mechanisms to enforce regulations, held by these Members to be a *prerequisite* for allowing the research to go forward; and an unwillingness to alienate large numbers of our fellow citizens who oppose this research on moral grounds.

Among Members who *disapprove* of cloning-for-biomedical-research, most oppose it permanently because they think it is immoral to create human embryos for purposes that are foreign to the embryos' own well-being and that necessarily require their destruction. Others oppose such cloning permanently because they hold that society (and not only the embryos) will suffer irreversible moral harm by crossing the boundary that allows nascent human life routinely to be treated as a natural resource. Some Members oppose permitting the practice because they fear that it will greatly increase the likelihood that cloning-to-produce-children will occur or because they think that a law banning only the transfer of a cloned embryo into a woman's uterus would be unenforceable. Some Members oppose the practice also because they think that the scientific case for proceeding has not yet met the burden of showing why this research is *necessary* and of sufficient importance to justify crossing the moral barrier of creating nascent human life for the purpose of experimentation.

(e) Were we to indicate where we stand on the ethical and prudential assessments of the two forms of human cloning, *each considered independently*, we would line up as follows:

	Permit Now (with Regulation)	Moratorium	Ban
To produce children	0	0	17
For biomedical research	7*	3	7

Where we stand on the *public policy options*—in which both cloning-to-produce-children and cloning-for-biomedical-research are *necessarily considered together*—we shall indicate below, in our recommendations.

(f) The Council notes that research on stem cells, both embryonic and adult, is still in its very early stages. Work with both embryonic and non-embryonic stem cells has led to some very promising results,† and it is impossible to predict which avenues of research will prove most successful in providing basic knowledge of disease processes and tools for regenerative medicine. It is likely that different diseases or research problems will require different approaches. The Council also notes that the possible benefits of cloning-for-biomedical-research are, at the present time, uncertain and undemonstrated. There is little evidence from animal experimentation to indicate, one way or the other, whether work with embryonic stem cells derived from *cloned* embryos offers *unique* benefits not otherwise available. Only further research can answer these questions. These uncertainties about

---

* This group includes some Members who would make the permission to proceed contingent upon the *prior* institution of strict regulations and a mechanism for enforcing them, and some Members who would allow the regulations to be developed as the research proceeds.

† The embryonic stem cells in these studies were obtained from *non-cloned* human embryos, produced by IVF.

the future should cut in two directions. They should temper claims of medical miracles just around the corner, placing a high demand for cautious accumulation of evidence. They should also temper assertions that biomedical researchers can pursue their goals without using human embryos because other approaches that are morally nonproblematic will surely prove successful.

(g) The Council notes, with special emphasis, that proposals to engage in cloning-for-biomedical-research necessarily endorse the creation of (cloned) human embryos *solely for the purpose of such research*. Public policy that specifically promoted this research would thus *explicitly and officially approve* crossing a moral boundary.*

(h) The Council also notes that, at the present time, human embryo research proceeds unregulated in commercial biotechnology companies and with local oversight in university-based laboratories (under the governance of institutional review boards [IRBs], whose oversight is generally stringent). In addition, federally funded research on human embryonic stem cell lines is now proceeding, under guidelines established by the National Institutes of Health pursuant to President Bush's decision of August 9, 2001. Any legislative action on human cloning, including cloning-for-biomedical-research, would not directly affect this other valuable research, including all research on embryonic stem cells derived from IVF embryos. In addition, a ban on cloning-for-biomedical-research would leave undisturbed the freedom that scientists (in the private sector) now have to create embryos solely for research by means of IVF, a practice that lacks official sanction and that has drawn public criticism but that is nonetheless legal (except in those few states that have banned this practice).

---

* The National Bioethics Advisory Commission recommended that federal agencies not fund research involving the derivation or use of human embryonic stem cells from embryos *made solely for research purposes* or *using SCNT*. (NBAC, *Ethical Issues in Human Stem Cell Research*, Vol. I, 1999, Recommendations 3 and 4, pp. 71-72.)

(i) Finally, in viewing congressional efforts in 1998 and in 2001-2002 to enact a legislative ban on human cloning, the Council notes the failure to enact a ban on cloning-to-produce-children—a ban that nearly everyone supports—because of irreconcilable differences between the supporters of cloning-for-biomedical-research and the opponents of any research that destroys (cloned) human embryos. Failure to prohibit cloning-to-produce-children, especially after protracted debate on the issue, amounts tacitly to public willingness to allow this practice to remain legal. We are accordingly interested in seeking a policy proposal that would, among other things, overcome this impasse.

Below are the two alternative proposals to which Council Members have given their support.

*   *   *

II. First Proposal

Ban on Cloning-to-Produce-Children, Moratorium on Cloning-for-Biomedical-Research (Policy Option 6 of Chapter Seven).

Call for a federal review of current and projected practices of human embryo research, preimplantation genetic diagnosis, genetic modification of human embryos and gametes, and related matters, with a view to recommending and shaping ethically sound policies for the entire field.

We recommend a congressionally enacted ban on all attempts at cloning-to-produce-children and a four-year national moratorium (a temporary ban) on human cloning-for-biomedical-research.* *These measures would apply everywhere in the United States and would govern the conduct of all researchers, physicians, institutions, or companies, whether or not they accept public funding. We also recommend that, during this moratorium, the federal government undertake a thoroughgoing review of present and projected practices of human embryo research, preimplantation genetic diagnosis, genetic modification of human embryos and gametes, and related matters, with a view to proposing, before the moratorium expires, an ethically acceptable public policy to govern these scientifically and medically promising but morally challenging activities. Several reasons converge to make this our recommended*

---

* Operationally, the legislation could address separately the two uses of cloning and define the prohibited acts as follows. Cloning I: the creation of a cloned human embryo by somatic cell nuclear transfer. Cloning II: the creation of a cloned human embryo, produced by somatic cell nuclear transfer, followed by transfer into a woman's (or animal's) uterus or into an artificial womb. It could then declare that: (1) Cloning I shall be unlawful for four years from the date of the enactment of this legislation. (2) Cloning II is hereby declared unlawful.

course of action at the present time. Members of the Council who support this recommendation do so for different reasons; some individual Members do not endorse all the concurring arguments given below.

A. Strengths of the Proposal

1. Bans Cloning-to-Produce-Children

The strong ethical verdict against cloning-to-produce-children, unanimous in this Council (and in Congress) and widely supported by the American people, is hereby translated into clear and strong legal proscription. The nation's moral conviction is expressed with force of law through the people's representatives. To be sure, such a ban (like any proscription) could be violated, but it could not be violated with impunity. By reflecting the pervasive moral judgment of the community, this ban would also serve as a source of moral instruction and a sign that we can exercise some control over the direction and use of biotechnology. Moreover, were we at this time to settle for a mere moratorium on cloning-to-produce-children, we might lose what may be our society's best chance to get a permanent ban on this practice before it occurs and to declare our opposition to the idea of designing and manufacturing our children. We would lose this precious opportunity to demonstrate that we are able to practice democratic self-rule regarding biotechnology and that we can establish firm guidelines for the moral practice of science and technology.

2. Provides a Highly Effective Means of Preventing Cloning-to-Produce-Children

The proposal's ban on all efforts to produce cloned children is a primary goal. The moratorium on cloning-for-biomedical-research (while desired by many for its own sake) would also provide an additional safeguard against cloning-to-produce-children during the next four years, beyond what would be available in a proposal that banned only the implantation of cloned embryos but left cloning-for-biomedical-research unregulated. By stopping all human cloning for four years, this proposal would prevent the creation of cloned embryos, thus decreasing the chances that anyone will be able to attempt to produce a cloned child. The moratorium would also permit time to explore other effective safeguards against this possibility that might be put in place should the moratorium not be reenacted after four years.

3. Calls for and Provides Time for Further Democratic Deliberation

A true national discourse on cloning-for-biomedical-research has not yet taken place. Certainly it has begun. But no consensus has been reached, no clear majority has appeared, and only in rare cases have the various parties to the debate acknowledged (as we have attempted to do in this report) that their opponents are also defending important and shared values. The matters at stake are too significant to be settled now—either by proceeding with the research with minimal delay or by banning the research outright—when the nation is so divided and when the implications of proceeding or not proceeding are as yet unclear. Under these circumstances, the proper attitude is modesty, caution, and moderation, expressed in a temporary ban to be revisited when time and democratic argumentation have clarified the matter. By allowing the debate and deliberation to continue, a moratorium would offer the following specific benefits:

(a) Seeking consensus on crossing a major moral boundary. To decide to create nascent human life expressly for the purpose of experimentation and use is to cross a significant moral boundary. It goes beyond permitting the use of extra embryos, created for reproductive purposes, that are stored in IVF clinics and otherwise destined for destruction. Yet the meaning and moral propriety of crossing such a boundary are today hotly contested. Many people believe that even the earliest stages of a new human life should be protected against such use and destruction and would oppose such a practice at any time. Many others favor permitting the practice, but only under conditions of strict governmental regulation that would guard against abuses and reflect measured respect for the embryonic life that is being sacrificed. Our society needs more time to explore the full moral significance of tak-

ing such a step, to debate the moral and practical issues involved, and to seek a national consensus—about *all* research on early human embryonic (and fetal) life (not just that formed through cloning techniques).

(b) Gaining needed scientific evidence. The moratorium on all human cloning will allow time for scientists to produce hard evidence from cloning research in animals and animal disease models—evidence not available today. Such evidence, if available, would support their present claims regarding the value of cloning-for-biomedical-research, both for understanding normal and disease processes and for finding new treatments. The moratorium will also provide time to see whether cloning research will be indispensable for these goals or whether there are equally fruitful but morally nonproblematic alternatives to cloning, (such as, for example, work with adult stem cells or multipotent adult progenitor cells or work that would solve the transplant rejection problem for tissues derived from ordinary embryonic stem cell lines).

(c) Promoting fuller and focused public debate, leading to a better-informed decision. For people who believe that the human embryo must not be violated, and who would therefore advocate a permanent ban on cloning-for-biomedical-research, this moratorium offers a partial step in what they deem to be the right direction, and an opportunity to make further progress through moral persuasion and political action. By preventing cloning-for-biomedical-research for a while, this proposal takes seriously their warnings of possible harms from allowing such research. But it also calls on them to make those warnings more concrete and convincing, by arguing their case *in the proper context of embryo research in general* and not just that of cloning. Meanwhile, those who now do (or later might) support cloning-for-biomedical-research would also find benefits in this moratorium. It would allow them the opportunity to make their full case and win over new supporters, to prepare the ground properly (using new scientific evidence) for agreement on the merits of research when the time to decide comes, and to devise safeguards against likely abuse and misuse. The public decision made after the moratorium expires would be

better informed and more fully considered as a result of such debate.

(d) Preserving a decent respect for the deep moral concerns of our fellow citizens. A large number of Americans, perhaps even a majority, hold that it is deeply immoral to create what they regard as new human life for the purposes of experimental research that involves the destruction of that life. We should be very reluctant to ride roughshod over these views and to practice contempt for our fellow citizens, especially for the sake of promised benefits that are at this point highly uncertain and speculative, and especially when the *necessity* of this approach to the treatment of disease has not been demonstrated and when the public debate has been so brief. A moratorium will enable us to respect and assess these moral concerns while we look to science to provide alternatives that do not require crossing this moral boundary. Should the community decide, after the ongoing deliberation made possible by the moratorium, to cross it, no group would have grounds to complain that its views had been treated with contempt. Also, we could have in the meantime established new boundaries and devised effective regulations that could give genuine assurance that additional and more problematic practices would be forestalled or avoided altogether.

4. Provides Time and Incentive to Develop Adequate Regulation Regarding Human Cloning

Because of the widespread concern to prevent cloning-to-produce-children, those who support cloning-for-biomedical-research bear the burden of devising and instituting adequate oversight and regulatory mechanisms that would effectively reduce the risk that embryos cloned for research might be used in efforts to produce cloned children. In addition, regulatory guidelines and mechanisms, devised and installed in advance, are called for regarding cloning-for-biomedical-research itself. Because everyone has a stake in how nascent human life is treated, serious efforts are necessary to protect the public interest. *Cloning-for-biomedical-research, if and when it is to be allowed, must be preceded by the formulation of proper rules and the institution of effective safeguards.*

Devising effective regulatory instruments takes time, and a moratorium could afford regulation proponents that time. Equally important, in the absence of a moratorium, *few proponents of the research would have much incentive to help institute an effective regulatory system.* And a governmental policy simply to withhold federal funding pending the development of a regulatory regimen would have no effect on the conduct of this research in the private sector. The following matters, at a minimum, would need to be considered by any serious program of regulation:

(a) Comprehensive scope. Regulations that would cover all cloning research, whether done with public or private funds, whether done in universities, private research institutes, assisted reproduction clinics, or biotech companies.

(b) Protections for egg donors. Regulations governing the safety and consent of the oocyte donors, with safeguards against improper inducements and exploitation of poor or otherwise vulnerable women.

(c) Transparency and accountability. Regulations permitting full public knowledge and scrutiny of what is being done with cloned embryos produced for research purposes.*

---

* Careful consideration should be given to the following matters: licensing requirements to engage in such research; accurate inventory and reporting of the numbers, uses, and fates of all cloned embryos; decisions about whether to permit the buying and selling of cloned human embryos; rules governing commerce or traffic in cloned human embryos, should it be allowed; patent law questions regarding cloned human embryos, blastocysts, and later stages of cloned human organisms; age and stage of embryonic development beyond which it would be impermissible to maintain and experiment upon cloned embryos; rules regarding the permissibility of growing cloned human embryos in animal hosts or artificial substitutes for a human or animal uterus; regulations concerning cloned human-animal chimeras (for example, human nuclei placed in animal oocytes); guidelines specifying the kinds of experiments that may be performed on the cloned embryos; guidelines regarding production levels and storage of cloned embryos; and, finally, effective institutional mechanisms—designed to prevent easy capture by cloning researchers or biotech companies—for monitoring cloning activities, enforcing the rules, and penalizing violators.

(d) Equal access to benefits. Guidelines to promote equal access to the medical benefits that flow from such research.

The very process of proposing such regulations would clarify the moral and prudential judgments involved in deciding whether and how to proceed with this research, as well as how cloning-for-biomedical research relates to other areas of embryological, reproductive, and genetic experimentation.

5. Calls for and Provides Time for a Comprehensive Review of the Entire Domain of Related Biotechnologies

A moratorium on cloning-for-biomedical-research would enable us to consider this activity in the larger context of research and technology in the areas of developmental biology and genetics. The practices of human embryo research and preimplantation genetic diagnosis are largely unregulated by the federal government, or regulated in a haphazard, uncoordinated way. These practices, along with those of assisted reproduction, are largely unstudied: we lack comprehensive knowledge about what is being done, with what success, at what risk, under what ethical guidelines, respecting which moral boundaries, subject to what oversight and regulation, and with what sanctions for misconduct or abuse. If we are to have wise public policy regarding these scientifically and medically promising but morally challenging activities, we need careful study and sustained public moral discourse on this general subject, and not only on specific narrowly defined pieces of the field. To achieve this goal, the moratorium here proposed should be accompanied by a concerted review of the entire field, with the aim of establishing permanent institutions to advise and shape federal policy in this arena.

The President's Council on Bioethics stands ready to undertake the preliminary steps of such a process and to provide advice on further steps. As part of our ongoing inquiry, we intend to continue to study various models of oversight and regulation of biomedical research and technology, both professional and governmental, that are used in the United States and abroad. As the necessary efforts will likely lead beyond the authority, scope, and perhaps also the duration of this advisory Council,* we shall be especially interested in recommendations for devising a more permanent national agency or institution, with broad oversight, advisory, and decision-making authority,† that could emerge before the expiration of the four-year moratorium here proposed. Such a body could provide much-needed understanding and national guidance on these vitally important subjects. Progress toward creating such a body would ratify and perpetuate the deliberative goals of the moratorium.

6. Provides Time to Garner Long-Term Respect and Support for Biomedical Research and to Reaffirm the Social Contract between Science and Society

A moratorium, rather than a lasting ban, signals a high regard for the value of biomedical research and an enduring concern for patients and families whose suffering such research may help alleviate. By providing time to consider whether and how regulations might govern research in this morally troubling area, the moratorium invites the scientific, medical, and industrial communities into the activities of devising boundaries that they themselves would willingly respect. Such responsible behavior of biomedical researchers would go a long way to protect them against a public backlash should some less responsible scientists or technologists engage in practices repugnant to community standards or should some of their experiments result in great harm to some human subjects. It would reaffirm the principle that science can progress while upholding the community's moral norms. It would reassure researchers that any public moral

---

* The President's Council on Bioethics is currently chartered through November 2003.

† In thinking about this process we think it will be helpful to consult the work of the Canadian Royal Commission on New Reproductive Technologies. The process by which that Commission arrived at its final conclusions, and its manner of presenting those conclusions (carefully taking into account voluminous public testimony and dissenting opinions) strike us as providing an excellent model worthy of study and, to the extent appropriate, emulation. The scope, principles, structure, and functions of the proposed Assisted Human Reproduction Agency of Canada seem to us worthy of special attention.

restrictions on their activities will be rare, strictly limited, and carefully drawn. It would reassure the community that there is to be no slippery slope toward significant interference with the progress of beneficial biomedical research, the treatment of human diseases, or the moral uses of biomedical technologies. Friction between scientists and the wider community, aggravated by precipitate decision, would be reduced. The community's moral support for science and biomedical technology would be reaffirmed, and, as a result, the *long-term* interests of patients, families, and the entire society could be better served.

B. Some Specifics for the Legislation

Drafting the legislation that would give effect to this proposal lies beyond the scope and competence of the Council. Yet the following considerations would seem to be indispensable for a well-drafted and effective statute.

1. Broad Coverage

The ban and moratorium should cover everyone, corporations as well as individuals, private as well as public institutions.

2. Narrowly Drafted

The statute should be very narrowly drafted, making sure that only the human cloning actions in question are proscribed, and indicating explicitly other research and assisted-reproduction practices that will not be in any way affected by the ban or moratorium.

3. Temporary

Regarding the moratorium on cloning-for-biomedical-research, in the event that Congress takes no further action after four years, the moratorium should lapse.

C. Conclusion

The proposal we recommend is, admittedly, a compromise, requiring some give on both sides of the national debate if it is to be enacted. But it is by no means merely a compromise. On the contrary, it is perfectly warranted by the state of public opinion and justified by the supreme value in our democracy of informed and deliberate decision in matters of great moment. If enacted, it would establish a permanent ban on cloning-to-produce-children, a practice that the nation overwhelmingly opposes. And it would not prematurely settle the equally important question of cloning-for-biomedical-research.

As already noted, this proposal accurately reflects the state of the public discussion of human cloning. There is broad agreement that cloning-to-produce-children should be banned, but there is deep disagreement and uncertainty regarding whether and how to proceed with cloning-for-biomedical-research. Such uncertainty calls for more discussion, more data, and more time—things a moratorium would provide. In proposing the combination of a ban on cloning-to-produce-children and a moratorium on cloning-for-biomedical-research, we do not imply that we hold one form of cloning to be worse than the other, but rather that the state of the public debate is such that a clearly-agreed-upon course of action presents itself in the one case, but more time and deliberation are called for in the other. Even some of us who see merit in proceeding with cloning-for-biomedical-research worry that cloning-for-biomedical-research may turn out to be morally worse than cloning-to-produce-children, at least in magnitude, especially should it lead to a routinized practice of embryo cultivation and the growth of nascent human life for body parts. But given the present state of the public discussion and the dearth of scientific evidence, the Council has not reached consensus on how to formulate a permanent policy on this matter at this moment, and the American people are apparently divided on the subject.

The proposal we have offered is not just an acknowledgement of the current lack of consensus. It is intended to advance the discussion toward an informed decision by forcing both sides to argue for their positions clearly and openly. A moratorium means that neither side would be free to cling to the status quo and avoid presenting its full case for public discussion.

On the one hand, the moratorium would permit and require the research community to provide the public with more information about the desirability and necessity of the research, and to indicate how it can go forward within proper limits and respectful of communal norms. It will also provide time and incentive for researchers to seek out and invest in alternative technological approaches that are morally nonproblematic. It may well be that when Congress revisits the issue after the moratorium expires, the facts on the ground may show no unique or compelling need for cloning-for-biomedical-research, and morally nonproblematic alternatives may have been discovered. Yet the ban on cloning-to-produce-children would remain in place regardless of what happens on the research front.

On the other hand, the moratorium would permit and require the community concerned about defending the inviolability of embryonic human life to continue the moral argument in the hope of persuading the broader society to desist. That argument, we point out, has to be about embryo research in general, and not just about cloned embryos in particular. With cloning-to-produce-children prohibited and hence off the table, the debate could focus honestly and fully on this central question.

We acknowledge the concerns raised by opponents of this proposal, who worry that even a four-year moratorium on cloning-for-biomedical-research cuts off urgently needed investigation, and that prominent scientists may be tempted to leave the United States for countries without such restrictions on cloning research. These are understandable worries, but we believe they are misplaced and are not sufficient to force an immediate decision on this subject.

First, the promise of this research is for now purely speculative, and no significant evidence from animal research has presented itself that might demonstrate that this (to many people) morally disquieting or objectionable practice is in fact *necessary* for the goals that researchers aim to serve, or that adult stem cells cannot provide equally good models for studying inherited diseases, or that other routes are not more effective in addressing the transplant rejection problem.

Second, there is more to this matter than scientific and medical progress. We ask proponents to recognize the moral hazards that such research would be unleashing. Treating nascent human life as a natural resource (or even, more respectfully, as a *human* resource to which we ought to feel indebted) is morally troubling, and there is a clear and present danger that it could lead us down a path where our reverence for life may be imperiled. We would therefore ask proponents of this research and the public-at-large to keep these moral concerns in mind as we try to develop a sound public policy for the whole area of embryo research. We think that the moratorium provides needed time to do this right.

Finally, while it is possible that a few scientists will leave the country if a moratorium is enacted, the vast majority will not. We have examples at the state and national levels (for instance, Michigan and Germany) where highly restrictive laws banning all human cloning have been enacted yet where the biotechnology industry is thriving. We have confidence that this robust field will continue to grow, including the area of stem cell research from sources other than cloned embryos (Indeed, several other countries, including France, Italy, Norway, South Korea, and Canada, permit work on embryonic stem cells but do not allow cloning-for-biomedical-research). Moreover, succumbing to the threat that some researchers might leave would not be a worthy way of making such a crucial moral decision. A scientist, like any other citizen, may choose to leave the United States for many different reasons. But there is no reason to assume that good scientists will not be able to work with and within the moral boundaries of the communities of which they are members and whose blessings and support they enjoy.

We believe that a permanent ban on cloning-to-produce-children coupled with a four-year moratorium on cloning-for-biomedical-research would be the best way for our society to express its firm position on the former, and to engage in a properly informed and open democratic deliberation on the latter. Moreover, combined with a systematic review at the federal level of the general field of embryo, reproductive, and genetic research and technology, this proposal would enable our society to think more comprehensively about how we should deal not just with human cloning but also with other vitally important areas of biotechnology. Ethical principles and boundaries need to be established; regulatory mechanisms need to be considered and devised; and ways must be found to give guidance to biomedical researchers and technological innovators so that beneficial research may proceed while upholding the moral and social norms of the community. The decision before us is of great moment and importance. Creating cloned embryos for *any* purpose requires crossing a major moral boundary, with grave risks and likely harms, and once we cross it there will be no turning back. Our society should take the time to do it right and to make a judgment that is well-informed and morally sound, respectful of strongly held views, and representative of the priorities and principles of the American people. We believe this proposal offers the best means of achieving these goals.

*   *   *

III. Second Proposal

Ban on Cloning-to-Produce-Children, with Regulation of the Use of Cloned Embryos for Biomedical Research (Policy Option 3 of Chapter Seven).

We recommend a congressionally enacted ban on all attempts at cloning-to-produce-children while preserving the freedom of cloning-for-biomedical-research. We recommend the establishment of a system of oversight and regulation that would permit cloning-for-biomedical-research to proceed promptly, but only under carefully prescribed limits. These measures would apply everywhere in the United States and would govern the conduct of all researchers, physicians, institutions, or companies, whether or not they accept public funding. In addition, we recommend that the federal government undertake a thoroughgoing review of present and projected practices of human embryo research. Several reasons converge to make this our recommended course of action at the present time. Members of the Council who support this recommendation do so for different reasons; some individual Members do not endorse all the concurring arguments given below.

A. Strengths of the Proposal

1. Bans Cloning-to-Produce-Children

The strong ethical verdict against cloning-to-produce-children, unanimous in this Council (and in Congress) and widely supported by the American people, is hereby translated into clear and strong legal proscription. The nation's moral conviction is expressed with force of law through the people's representatives. To be sure, such a ban (like any proscription) could be violated, but it could not be violated with impunity. By reflecting the pervasive moral judgment of the community, this ban would also serve as a source of moral instruction and a sign that we can exercise some control over the direction and use of biotechnology. Moreover, were we at this time to settle for a mere moratorium on cloning-to-produce-children, we might lose what may be our society's best chance to get a permanent ban on this practice before it occurs and to declare our opposition to the idea of designing and manufacturing our children. We would lose this precious opportunity to demonstrate that we are able to practice democratic self-rule regarding biotechnology and that we can establish firm guidelines for the moral practice of science and technology.[*]

2. Provides an Effective Means of Preventing Cloning-to-Produce-Children

Statutory prohibition on the transfer of a cloned human embryo to a woman's uterus, backed by heavy penalties, would provide a sufficient deterrent for anyone contemplating cloning-to-produce-children. Cloned embryos created for research could, it is true, possibly get into the hands of those who would attempt to use them to produce cloned children. But the regulatory mechanisms and guidelines governing cloning-for-biomedical-research, provided for by this proposal (see below), will greatly minimize the likelihood of such an occurrence. And anyone who attempted to clone a child could not claim the credit for any successes without incurring prosecution. Even if slightly less foolproof than a ban that also blocked the creation of cloned embryos, this is a sufficiently effective means for preventing cloning-to-produce-children.

3. Approves Cloning-for-Biomedical-Research and Permits It to Proceed without Substantial Delay

Here is the major benefit to be obtained from this proposal (benefits foreclosed by the First Proposal). This proposal would provide clear congressional endorsement of the importance of proceeding with cloning-for-biomedical-research. This potentially very valuable research, promising for all the reasons enu-

---

[*] On this point and some others to follow, this policy proposal is identical to the First Proposal. To indicate this fact, the earlier argument will sometimes be repeated in this Second Proposal verbatim. We do so for symmetry and balance, and to allow each proposal to be read as a self-contained unit, without relying on the other.

merated in Chapter Six, Part III ("The Moral Case for Cloning-for-Biomedical-Research") could now go forward without substantial delay using *human* cloned embryos and the stem cells and tissues derived therefrom. Uncertainty about the potential of this research can only be overcome by doing the research. It will be critically important to compare directly the advantages and disadvantages of adult stem cells, embryonic stem cells from IVF blastocysts, and embryonic stem cells from cloned blastocysts side by side in the same laboratory. Regardless of how much time we allow, no amount of experimentation with animal models could provide the essential and urgently needed understanding of *human* diseases. Moreover, the special and possibly unique benefits of stem cell research using *cloned* embryos (see Chapter Six, Part III) cannot be obtained using embryos produced by in vitro fertilization. The possible benefits to potentially millions of patients are so great that we think they should be pursued as soon as possible (under proper guidelines and regulations; see next point). While not disturbing the current policy on embryo research (which permits federal funding for research only on certain designated stem cell lines), this proposal explicitly eschews federal legal bans on new approaches to the revolutionary possibilities of regenerative medicine.

4. Establishes Necessary Protections against Possible Misuses and Abuses, Thus Paying the Respect Owed to Embryos Sacrificed in the Research

Unlike those human cloning bills, recently considered by Congress, that would permit cloning-for-biomedical-research, this proposal takes seriously the special respect owed to nascent human life as well as the moral hazards involved in this research, and it proposes concrete steps to prevent or minimize them. While such regulation will not satisfy those who believe that all such research is morally wrong, it will give concrete expression to our view that human embryos are never merely a *natural* resource, and that the special respect owed to them as *human* resources must be reflected in limits on what we may do with them. In addition, such regulation may succeed in assuaging everyone's worst fears about where this research might lead.[*]

Because of our concern to prevent cloning-to-produce-children, we call for adequate oversight and regulatory mechanisms to effectively reduce the risk that embryos cloned for research might be used in efforts to produce cloned children. In addition, we welcome regulatory guidelines and mechanisms, devised in advance, regarding cloning-for-biomedical-research itself. We agree that everyone has a stake in how nascent human life is treated, and that therefore serious efforts are necessary to protect the public interest. And although we want now to approve cloning-for-bio-medical-research, we agree that it shall not go forward in the absence of appropriate regulations and effective mechanisms for enforcing them.

Although this is not the place to draft legislation, the regulatory mechanisms we favor would be based on the following principles:

(a) Prevent cloned embryos from being used to initiate pregnancies. To do this, regulations must register, inventory, and track the fate of individual cloned embryos; prohibit the shipping or sale of cloned embryos (but not stem cells or other tissues or products derived from these embryos).

(b) Provide enforceable ethical guidelines for the use of cloned embryos for research. To do this, regulations must license and conduct prior review of all research involving cloned human embryos; set a definite time limit and developmental stage beyond which a cloned human embryo may not be grown, either in vitro or in vivo (we suggest fourteen days, or the formation of the primitive streak); prohibit the transfer of a cloned human embryo into the womb (or other gestational environment) of a human being or an ani-

---

[*] See Position Number One of "The Moral Case for Cloning-for-Biomedical-Research" in Chapter Six and the discussion of Policy Option 3 in Chapter Seven for the details of the moral hazards and how specific regulations can deal with them.

mal (or into an artificial equivalent of the same) for research purposes; and provide strong penalties to deter unlicensed or impermissible research.

(c) Protect the adult participants in this research. To do this, regulations must establish clear regulations for the protection of any human egg donors; set rules for financial compensation for egg donation; and establish other relevant measures designed to protect against the exploitation of women.

(d) Promote equal access to the medical benefits that flow from this research. To do this, guidelines must be developed that will keep down costs of medical therapies made available through this research, which would have been explicitly sanctioned by the community to serve the health needs of all.

5. Who Should Regulate This?

Whether done by an existing agency or a new one devised for this purpose, the regulatory authority should include scientists, physicians, and representatives of the biotechnology and pharmaceutical industries, but also lawyers, ethicists, humanists, clergy, and members of the public. In its composition and in its activities, every effort should be made to avoid even the appearance of conflict of interest, to prevent capture by special interests, and to ensure that the public's moral concerns are fully addressed in the devising of the regulations. A special Cloning Research Review Board, appointed by the President, might be one way to ensure high visibility and accountability.

6. Calls for a Comprehensive Review of the Entire Domain of Embryo Research

The ethical and policy issues regarding cloning-for-biomedical-research deserve to be considered in the context of all human embryo research. Regulatory mechanisms for cloning-for-biomedical research should be part of a larger regulatory program governing all research involving human embryos. To achieve this goal, we recommend that the federal government undertake a thorough-going review of present and projected practices of human embryo research, with the aim of establishing appropriate institutions to advise and shape federal policy in this arena.

B. Some Specifics for the Legislation

Drafting the legislation that would give effect to this proposal lies beyond the scope and competence of the Council. Yet the following considerations would seem to be indispensable for a well-drafted and effective statute.

1. Broad Coverage

The ban on cloning-to-produce-children, as well as the regulations devised for cloning-for-bio-medical-research, should cover everyone, corporations as well as individuals, private as well as public institutions.

2. Narrowly Drafted

The statute should be very narrowly drafted, making sure that only the human cloning actions in question are proscribed and indicating explicitly other research and assisted-reproduction practices that will not be in any way affected by the ban or regulations.

C. Conclusion

This recommendation is above all grounded in the importance of not needlessly foreclosing or delaying a promising avenue of medical research. Permitting cloning-for-biomedical-research now, while governing it through a prudent and sensible regulatory regime, is the most appropriate way to allow this important research to proceed while ensuring that abuses are prevented. Combined with a firm ban on the transfer of cloned embryos into a woman's uterus, as we have recommended, such a policy would provide the balance of freedom and protection, medical progress and respect for moral standards, always sought in a free society. Most important, it would leave open and endorse an important new avenue of research that might help alleviate the suffering of millions of our fellow citizens.

We respect and recognize the concerns of many in the public and in this Council regarding cloning-for-biomedical-research, especially about the need for further deliberation and the necessary safeguards to prevent cloning-to-produce-children. But we do not believe that our proposal forecloses continued deliberation. On the contrary, the public process of designing a system to regulate cloning-for-biomedical-research is likely to generate public discussion about the difficult ethical issues posed by embryo research in general.

First, the ban we propose on cloning-to-produce-children would be a strong deterrent against a practice that the nation overwhelmingly opposes. By stopping, with the force of law, the transfer of cloned embryos into a uterus, this ban would effectively prevent the cloning of children. Like any law, the ban we propose could be violated, but so too could a more comprehensive ban on all cloning of embryos. Moreover, we believe that the sort of regulatory mechanisms we have proposed here would provide sufficient protection against the implantation of cloned embryos. Research scientists and fertility specialists are not out to break the law or violate the moral norms of their communities. They can in general be relied upon to abide by the ban we have proposed, and those who violate it can be penalized.

Second, we believe that the regulatory system we have proposed would address those concerns specific to cloning-for-biomedical-research itself. We do not discount these concerns. The moral seriousness of working with nascent human life and the larger public concern about where this research may lead make it imperative, even as a matter of enlightened self-interest, for the research community to welcome and participate in the regulation of this research. Because the issues at stake are not just those of safety and efficacy, but moral and social ones as well, the participation of other citizens in these decisions is entirely appropriate. Cooperation with the broader community in this matter of public moral concern can only advance the relations between science and technology and the broader society.

Third, we do not believe that cloning-for-biomedical-research is the place to settle the more general question of research on human embryos. That is why we have proposed that the federal government review in a systematic way the general field of embryo research, with an eye to devising a possible set of general policies or institutions. In the meantime, it seems inappropriate to halt promising embryo research in one arena (cloned embryos) while it proceeds essentially unregulated in others. A sensible system of regulation will allow this important research to continue safely, while the nation considers a possible general policy on all embryo research.

Last, in answer to the specific concern that our proposal may put the government in the position of mandating the destruction of human embryos, we point out that those who would be producing the cloned embryos for research would have absolutely no intention of keeping them alive beyond the limits needed for the research. Hence there would be no occasion when governmental interference might be called for to compel unwilling researchers to destroy the cloned embryos. Strictly speaking, it would be the researchers, not government officials, who would be responsible for the destruction of the embryos; the government would not be requiring anything that was not already implicit in the research activity itself. True, the government, by enacting this legislation, would be accepting the use of cloned embryos for research, but it would be doing so fully mindful of the moral cost, for very good reason and under strict guidelines.

We therefore believe that the legitimate concerns about human cloning expressed throughout this report are sufficiently addressed by a ban on cloning-to-produce-children and the regulation of cloning-for-biomedical-research. And we believe that the nation should affirm and support the responsible effort to find treatments and cures that might help ameliorate or thwart diseases and disabilities that shorten life, limit activity (often severely), and cause great suffering for the afflicted and their families. Finding a way to support such valuable research while pre-serving moral standards is the challenge that confronts the fed-eral government and the American public in the matter of clon-ing. We believe our approach offers the best means of achieving that goal.

*   *   *

IV. Recommendation

After extensive deliberation, Members of the Council have coalesced around the two policy proposals, as follows:

The following ten Members of the Council form a majority in support of the First Proposal: Rebecca S. Dresser, Francis Fukuyama, Robert P. George, Mary Ann Glendon, Alfonso Gómez-Lobo, William B. Hurlbut, Leon R. Kass, Charles Krauthammer, Paul McHugh, Gilbert C. Meilaender.

The following seven Members of the Council form a minority in support of the Second Proposal: Elizabeth H. Blackburn, Daniel W. Foster, Michael S. Gazzaniga, William F. May, Janet D. Rowley, Michael J. Sandel, James Q. Wilson.

Glossary of Terms

Asexual reproduction
Reproduction *not* initiated by the union of oocyte and sperm. Reproduction in which all (or virtually all) the genetic material of an offspring comes from a single progenitor.

Blastocyst
Name used for an organism at the blastocyst stage of development.

Blastocyst stage
An early stage in the development of embryos, when (in mammals) the embryo is a spherical body comprising an inner cell mass that will become the fetus surrounded by an outer ring of cells that will become part of the placenta.

Cloned embryo
An embryo arising from the somatic cell nuclear transfer process as contrasted with an embryo arising from the union of an egg and sperm.

Cloning
- *Cloning-to-produce-children*—Production of a cloned human embryo, formed for the (proximate) purpose of initiating a pregnancy, with the (ultimate) goal of producing a child who will be genetically virtually identical to a currently existing or previously existing individual.
- *Cloning-for-biomedical-research*—Production of a cloned human embryo, formed for the (proximate) purpose of using it in research or for extracting its stem cells, with the (ultimate) goals of gaining scientific knowledge of

229

normal and abnormal development and of developing cures for human diseases.

- *Gene (molecular) cloning*—Isolation and characterization of DNA segments coding for proteins (genes) using carrier pieces of DNA called vectors.
- *Human cloning*—The asexual reproduction of a new human organism that is, at all stages of development, genetically virtually identical to a currently existing, or previously existing, human being.

Chromosomes

Structures inside the nucleus of a cell, made up of long pieces of DNA coated with specialized cell proteins, that are duplicated at each cell division. Chromosomes thus transmit the genes of the organism from one generation to the next.

Cytoplasmic

Located inside the cell but not in the nucleus.

Diploid

Refers to the chromosome number in a cell, distinct for each species (forty-six in human beings).

Diploid human cell

A cell having forty-six chromosomes.

Embryo

1. The developing organism from the time of fertilization until significant differentiation has occurred, when the organism becomes known as a fetus.
2. An organism in the early stages of development.

Enucleated egg

An egg cell whose nucleus has been removed or destroyed.

Epigenetic modification

The process of turning genes on and off during cell differentiation. It may be accomplished by changes in (a) DNA methylation, (b) the assembly of histone proteins into nucleosomes, and (c) remodeling of chromosome-associated proteins such as linker histones.

Epigenetic reprogramming

The process of removing epigenetic modifications of chromosomal DNA, so that genes whose expression was turned off during embryonic development and cell differentiation become active again. In cloning, epigenetic reprogramming of the donor cell chromosomal DNA is used to reactivate the complex program of gene expression and repression required for embryonic development.

Eugenics

An attempt to alter (with the aim of improving) the genetic constitution of future generations.

Gamete

A reproductive cell (egg or sperm).

Haploid human cell

A cell such as an egg or sperm that contains only twenty-three chromosomes.

Infertility

The inability to conceive a child through sexual intercourse.

In vitro fertilization (IVF)

The union of an egg and sperm, where the event takes place outside the body and in an artificial environment (the literal meaning of "in vitro" is "in glass"; for example, in a test tube).

Mitochondria

Small energy-producing organelles inside of cells. Mitochondria give rise to other mitochondria by copying their small piece of mitochondrial DNA and passing one copy of the DNA along to each of the two resulting mitochondria.

Moral status

The standing of a being or entity in relation to other moral agents or individuals. To have moral status is to be an entity toward which human beings, as moral agents, have or can have moral obligations.

Multipotent cell

A cell that can produce several different types of differentiated cells.

Nucleus

An organelle, present in almost all types of cells, which contains the chromosomes.

Nuclear transfer

Transferring the nucleus with its chromosomal DNA from one (donor) cell to another (recipient) cell. In cloning, the recipient is a human egg cell and the donor cell can be any one of a number of different adult tissue cells.

Oocyte

Egg.

Organism

Any living individual animal considered as a whole.

Parthenogenesis

A form of nonsexual reproduction in which eggs are subjected to electrical shock or chemical treatment in order to initiate cell division and embryonic development.

Pluripotent

A cell that can give rise to many different types of differentiated cells.

Somatic cell (human)

A diploid cell containing forty-six chromosomes obtained or derived from a living or deceased human body at any stage of development.

Somatic cell nuclear transfer (SCNT)

Transfer of the nucleus from a donor somatic cell into an enucleated egg to produce a cloned embryo.

Stem cells

Stem cells are undifferentiated multipotent precursor cells that are capable both of perpetuating themselves as stem cells and of undergoing differentiation into one or more specialized types of cells.

Totipotent

A cell with an unlimited developmental potential, such as the zygote and the cells of the very early embryo, each of which is capable of giving rise to (1) a complete adult organism and all of its tissues and organs, as well as (2) the fetal portion of the placenta.

Zygote

The diploid cell that results from the fertilization of an egg cell by a sperm cell.

Bibliography

Appleyard, B. *Brave New Worlds: Staying Human in the Genetic Future*. New York: Viking, 1998.

Bahn, S., et al. "Neuronal target genes of the neuron-restrictive silencer factor in neurospheres derived from fetuses with Down's syndrome: A gene expression study." *The Lancet*, 359: 310-315, 2002.

Baird, P., chair, Royal Commission on New Reproductive Technologies. Presentation at the June 2002 meeting of the President's Council on Bioethics, Washington, D.C. Transcript available on the Council's web site at www.bioethics.gov.

Belmont Report. The National Commission for the Protection of Human Subjects of Biomedical and Behavioral Research. *The Belmont Report: Ethical Principles and Guidelines for the Protection of Human Subjects of Research*. Bethesda, MD: Government Printing Office, 1978.

Briggs, R., and T.J. King. "Transplantation of living nuclei from blastula cells into enucleated frog's eggs." *Proceedings of the National Academy of Sciences* (USA), 38: 455-463, 1952.

Brown, D. "Human Clone's Birth Predicted; Delivery Outside U.S. May Come By 2003, Researcher Says." *The Washington Post*, 16 May 2002, A8.

Bush, G.W. "Remarks on Human Cloning Legislation." *Weekly Compilation of Presidential Documents*, 38, no. 15: 608-610, 10 April 2002.

Chesne, P., et al. "Cloned rabbits produced by nuclear transfer from adult somatic cells."
Nature Biotechnology, 20: 366-369, 2002.

Cibelli, J.B., et al. "Somatic cell nuclear transfer in humans: Pronuclear and early embryonic development." *e-biomed: The Journal of Regenerative Medicine*, 2: 25-31, 2001.

Cibelli, J.B., et al. "The health profile of cloned animals." *Nature Biotechnology*, 20:13-14, 2002a.

Cibelli, J.B., et al. "Parthenogenetic stem cells in nonhuman primates." *Science*, 295: 819, 2002b.

Clinton, W.J. "Memorandum on the Prohibition on Federal Funding for Cloning of Human Beings." *Weekly Compilation of Presidential Documents*, 33, no. 10: 281, 4 March 1997.

Code of Federal Regulations (CFR) Title 45, Part 46.111(a)(2).

Fletcher, J. *The Ethics of Genetic Control: Ending Reproductive Roulette.* New York: Anchor Books, 1974.

Fukuyama, F. *Our Posthuman Future: Consequences of the Biotechnology Revolution.* New York: Farrar, Straus and Giroux, 2002.

Gaylin, W. "The Frankenstein Myth Becomes a Reality—We Have the Awful Knowledge to Make Exact Copies of Human Beings." *New York Times Magazine*, 5 March 1972.

Gurdon, J.B. "The developmental capacity of nuclei taken from intestinal epithelium cells of feeding tadpoles." *Journal of Embryology and Experimental Morphology*, 10: 622-640, 1962.

Hagell, P., and P. Brundin. "Cell survival and clinical outcome following intrastriatal transplantation in Parkinson's disease." *Journal of Neuropathology and Experimental Neurology*, 60: 741-752, 2001.

Hall, C.T. "UCSF Admits Human Clone Research; Work to Duplicate Embryos for Medical Purposes on Hold." *San Francisco Chronicle*, 25 May 2002, A1.

Hansen, M., et al. "The Risk of Major Birth Defects after Intracytoplasmic Sperm Injection and In Vitro Fertilization." *New England Journal of Medicine*, 346: 725-730, 2002.

Helsinki Declaration. 18th World Medical Association General Assembly. *Ethical Principles for Medical Research Involving Human Subjects*. Helsinki, 1964 (amended 1975, 1983, 1989, 1996, 2000).

Hemingway, E. *The Old Man and the Sea*. New York: Simon & Schuster, 1996.

Hill, J.R. "Placental defects in nuclear transfer (cloned) animals." Paper presented at *Workshop: Scientific and Medical Aspects of Human Cloning*, National Academy of Sciences, Washington, D.C., 7 August 2001.

Hill J.R., et al. "Clinical and pathologic features of cloned transgenic calves and fetuses (13 case studies)." *Theriogenology*, 8: 1451-1465, 1999.

Huxley, A. *Brave New World*. New York: Harper Perennial, 1998.

Jaenisch, R., and I. Wilmut. "Don't clone humans!" *Science*, 291: 5513, 2001.

Jiang, Y., et al. "Pluripotency of mesenchymal stem cells derived from adult marrow." *Nature*, 418: 41-49, 2002.

Jonas, H. "Philosophical Reflections on Experimenting With Human Subjects." In *Readings on Ethical and Social Issues in Biomedicine*, edited by Richard W. Wertz. Englewood Cliffs, N.J.: Prentice-Hall, 1973.

Kass, L. "Making Babies—The New Biology and the 'Old' Morality." *The Public Interest*, No. 26: 18-56, Winter 1972.

Kass, L. "The Wisdom of Repugnance." *The New Republic*, 2 June 1997, 17-26.

Kass, L. "Preventing a Brave New World: Why We Should Ban Human Cloning Now." *The New Republic*, 21 May 2001, 30-39.

Kass, L. "The Meaning of Life—in the Laboratory." *The Public Interest*, No. 146: 45-46, Winter 2002.

Kim, J.-H., et al. "Dopamine neurons derived from embryonic stem cells function in an animal model of Parkinson's disease." *Nature*, 418: 50-56, 2002.

Kluger, J. "Here Kitty Kitty!" *Time*, 159(8), 25 February 2002 (issued online February 17, 2002).

Kolata, G. *Clone: The Road to Dolly and the Path Ahead.* New York: Morrow and Company, 1998.

Kolata, G. "In Cloning, Failure Far Exceeds Success." *New York Times*, 11 December 2001, D1.

Kristol, W., and E. Cohen. *The Future Is Now.* Lanham, MD: Rowman and Littlefield, 2002.

Lanza, R.P., et al. "Human therapeutic cloning." *Nature Medicine*, 5: 975-977, 1999.

Lanza, R.P., et al. "Cloned cattle can be healthy and normal." *Science*, 294: 1893-1894, 2001.

Lanza, R.P., et al. "Generation of histocompatible tissues using nuclear transplantation." *Nature Biotechnology*, 2: 689-696, 2002.

Lederberg, J. "Experimental Genetics and Human Evolution." *The American Naturalist*, 100: 519-536, September-October 1966.

Leggett, K., and A. Regalado. "China Stem Cell Research Surges as Western Nations Ponder Ethics." *Wall Street Journal*, 6 March 2002, A1.

Macklin, R. Testimony before the National Bioethics Advisory Commission, March 14, 1997. Transcript available at www.georgetown.edu/research/nrcbl/nbac/.

National Academy of Sciences (NAS). *Scientific and Medical Aspects of Human Reproductive Cloning.* Washington, D.C.: National Academy Press, 2002.

National Bioethics Advisory Commission (NBAC). *Cloning Human Beings.* Bethesda, MD: Government Printing Office, 1997.

National Bioethics Advisory Commission (NBAC). *Ethical Issues in Human Stem Cell Research.* Bethesda, MD: Government Printing Office, 1999.

National Institutes of Health (NIH). Ad Hoc Group of Consultants to the Advisory Committee to the Director (Human Embryo Research Panel). *Report.* Bethesda, MD: Government Printing Office, 1994.

National Research Council/Institute of Medicine (NRC/IOM). *Stem Cells and the Future of Regenerative Medicine.* Washington, D.C.: National Academy Press, 2001.

Nuremberg Report. *Trials of War Criminals before the Nuremberg Military Tribunals under Control Council Law No. 10. Vol. 2, pp. 181-182.* Washington, D.C.: Government Printing Office, 1949.

Nussbaum, M., and C.R. Sunstein. *Clones and Clones: Facts and Fantasies about Human Cloning.* New York: Norton, 1998.

Ogonuki, N., et al. "Early death of mice cloned from somatic cells." *Nature Genetics,* 30: 253-254, 2002.

Osler, W. "Chauvinism in Medicine." In *Aequanimitas, with Other Addresses to Medical Students, Nurses and Practitioners of Medicine.* Philadelphia: Blakiston, 1943.

Outka, G. "The Ethics of Human Stem Cell Research." Paper presented at the April 2002 meeting of the President's Council on Bioethics, posted at the Council's web site at www.bioethics.gov. A slightly revised version of this article appears in the *Kennedy Institute of Ethics Journal,* 12, No. 2: 175-213, 2002.

President's Commission for the Study of Ethical Problems in Medicine and Biomedical and Behavioral Research. *Splicing Life: A Report on the Social and Ethical Issues of Genetic Engineering with Human Beings.* Washington, D.C.: Government Printing Office, 1982.

Ramsey, P. *Fabricated Man: The Ethics of Genetic Control.* New Haven: Yale University Press, 1970.

Regalado, A. "Only Nine Lives for Kitty? Not if She Is Cloned." *Wall Street Journal,* 14 February 2002, B1.

Reyes, M., et al. "Origin of endothelial progenitors in human postnatal bone marrow." *Journal of Clinical Investigation,* 109: 337-346, 2002.

Rideout III, W.M., et al. "Nuclear cloning and epigenetic reprogramming of the genome." *Science,* 293: 1093-1098, 2001.

Rideout III, W.M., et al. "Correction of a genetic defect by nuclear transplantation and combined cell and gene therapy." *Cell,* 109: 17-27, 2002.

Rimington, M., E. Simons, and K. Ahuja. "Counseling patients undergoing ovarian stimulation about the risks of ovarian hyperstimulation syndrome," *Human Reproduction,* 14: 2921-2922, 1999.

Robertson, J.A. "A Ban on Cloning and Cloning Research Is Unjustified." Testimony before the National Bioethics Advisory Commission, 14 March 1997.

Rorvik, D. *In His Image: The Cloning of a Man.* New York: J.B. Lippincott, 1978.

Rougier, N., and Z. Werb. "Minireview: Parthenogenesis in mammals." *Molecular Reproduction and Development,* 59: 468-474, 2001.

Saad, L. "Cloning Humans Is a Turn-Off to Most Americans." *Gallup Poll Analyses,* 16 May 2002.

Shamblott, M.J., et al. "Derivation of pluripotent stem cells from cultured human primordial germ cells." *Proceedings of the National Academy of Science* (USA), 95: 13726-13731, 1998.

Shin, T., et al. "A cat cloned by nuclear transplantation." *Nature,* 415: 859, 2002.

Spemann, H. *Embryonic Development and Induction.* New Haven: Yale University Press, 1938.

Stent, G. "Molecular biology and metaphysics" *Nature,* 248: 779-781, 1974.

Supreme Court of the United States. *Eisenstadt v. Baird,* 405 U.S. 438, 1972.

Thomson, J.A., et al. "Embryonic stem cell lines derived from human blastocysts." *Science,* 282: 1145-1147, 1998.

Tribe, L. "On Not Banning Cloning for the Wrong Reasons." In M. Nussbaum and C.R. Sunstein, *Clones and Clones: Facts and Fantasies about Human Cloning.* New York: Norton, 1998.

Vogelstein, B., et al. "Please don't call it cloning!" *Science,* 295: 1237, 2002.

Wakayama, T., et al. "Cloning of mice to six generations." *Nature*, 407: 318-319, 2000.

Wakeley, K., and E. Grendys. "Reproductive technologies and risk of ovarian cancer." *Current Opinion in Obstetrics and Gynecology*, 12: 43-47, 2000.

Watson, J. "Moving Toward the Clonal Man." *The Atlantic Monthly*, May 1971.

Watson, J. Testimony before the Committee on Science and Astronautics, U. S. House of Representatives, Ninety-Second Congress, January 26, 27, and 28, 1971.

Weiss, R. "Human Cloning Bid Stirs Experts' Anger; Problems in Animal Cases Noted." *The Washington Post*, 11 April 2001, A1.

Weiss, R. "Stem Cell Transplant Works in Calif. Case, Parkinson's Traits Largely Disappear." *The Washington Post*, 9 April 2002, A8.

Wilmut, I. "Application of animal cloning data to human cloning." Paper presented at *Workshop: Scientific and Medical Aspects of Human Cloning*, National Academy of Sciences, Washington, D.C., 7 August 2001.

Wilmut, I. et al. "Viable offspring derived from fetal and adult mammalian cells." *Nature*, 385: 810-813, 1997.

Wilson, J.Q. "On Abortion." *Commentary*, 97, No. 1: 21ff, 1994.

APPENDIX

Appendix

Personal Statements

The eight chapters, plus Bibliography and Glossary of Terms, constitute the official body of this report. Though it contains expressed differences of opinion, especially in Chapters Six and Eight, it stands as the work of the entire Council. In the interest of contributing further to public discussion of the issues, and of enabling individual Members of the Council to speak in their own voice on one or another aspect of this report, we offer in this Appendix personal statements from those Members who have elected to submit them:

Elizabeth H. Blackburn, Ph.D., D.Sc.
Rebecca S. Dresser, J.D., M.S.
Daniel W. Foster, M.D.
Michael S. Gazzaniga, Ph.D.
Robert P. George, D.Phil., J.D. (joined by Alfonso Gómez-Lobo, Ph.D.)
William B. Hurlbut, M.D.
Charles Krauthammer, M.D.
Paul McHugh, M.D.
William F. May, Ph.D.
Gilbert C. Meilaender, Ph.D.
Janet D. Rowley, M.D., D.Sc.
Michael J. Sandel, D.Phil.
James Q. Wilson, Ph.D.

* * *

Statement of Professor Blackburn

Why a Moratorium on Cloning-for-Biomedical-Research Is Not the Way to Proceed

There are several reasons why a moratorium on cloning-for-biomedical-research (SCNT) is not a logical or productive direction in which to proceed.

The goal of a moratorium is to wait until something happens, then make a decision. For a moratorium on SCNT (cloning-for-biomedical-research), waiting would have several consequences that I do not believe reflect the spirit of much of the Council's opinion.

First, during any such proposed moratorium, patients will continue to have currently incurable diseases—for which there is now no hope of alleviation—and many will continue to die of them. Second, a moratorium is used to gain more information. It may sound tempting to impose a moratorium to get more information, since, despite very promising results, it is true, at this early stage of the research, that we still know only a little. But that information can *only* be gained by performing the same research that the moratorium proposes to halt.

It has been proposed that other kinds of research will provide such answers. One cannot find out the answers about oranges by doing all the research on apples. Some kinds of research on apples will be useful, because it will provide information about generalities that apply to fruit in general. But diseases are very specific, and humans are very specific. They share overarching features with other animals, but the very nature of disease is to be particular. Thus, diabetes research does not apply to Parkinson's research.

Furthermore, it has been proposed that the needed information can be gained from research in animal models. However, it is of crucial importance to be aware that human diseases are different, in certain specific ways, from their counterpart models in animals. This is the case just as the course of development in a mouse has overarching similarities to, yet at the same time startling and highly specific differences from, the course of development of a human. Hence, animal models, while invaluable up to a point, cannot provide the needed information for understanding and treating a human disease.

Currently, there are excess in vitro fertilization embryos, and it has been proposed that biomedical research on these, if allowed by their parents and those responsible for them, would be adequate for obtaining the types of information that could be gained from research that involves SCNT. But first, these excess embryos represent only a limited set of genetic backgrounds. They do not represent the wide diversity of genetic and ethnic groups that will be needed if the fruits of this research are to be available to all. Second, the limited set of available excess IVF embryos would not, of course, represent the very genotypes of perhaps greatest interest: those representing the diseases that are the rightful subject of research involving SCNT. A final point concerns why these embryos are in excess. It is not only to attempt to ensure success of IVF, but also, in current IVF practice, these excess embryos are more often the ones that were judged by the IVF clinic professionals as appearing less likely to develop well—which is why they were not chosen for implantation in the first place. If they have a higher chance of abnormality, this is not the group of embryos that is ideal for obtaining the best, most relevant information about development and disease.

SCNT-derived stem cells could provide other crucial information, in a way impossible for excess in-vitro-fertilized-embryo-derived stem cells. Researchers could address, in a clear and experimentally controlled way, a key unknown issue about the therapeutic value of stem cell use for regenerative medicine: the immune rejection issue. There are excellent in vitro investigations that could cast a lot of much needed light on this area, and could be done only with cells derived from the same genetic background—i.e., using stem cells from SCNT. Again, this cannot be done with animal models alone, which have been the only source of information on this topic to date, because we know that animal models are not complete models for many particular biological questions in humans.

In sum, reliance on excess IVF embryos would severely hobble efforts to gain the information that is needed to be able to judge the promise of cloning-for-biomedical-research. Further, the use of IVF embryos in no way facilitates the most immediately promising areas of SCNT research, which involve not tissue transplantation but rather the development of laboratory tissue that has been grown from somatic cells with known genetic mutations that are needed for study and for testing of new pharmaceutical interventions.

Hence, a moratorium, imposed in order to wait for more information that will give us a better informed set of facts from which to proceed, is logically flawed.

The President's Council on Bioethics currently is proposing two possible policy recommendations. Both would ban cloning-to-produce-children. One proposal is to proceed with cloning-for-biomedical-research (SCNT) with appropriate regulations; the other is to put it under a four-year moratorium. I support the former proposal.

Some have called for a moratorium pending development of elaborate regulatory innovations, such as the creation of a new government body to oversee all this research. Unfortunately, such regulations might well never emerge, allowing opponents of research to accomplish by administrative delay what they have been unable to accomplish through legislation, that is, a de facto ban on SCNT research. Furthermore, these proposals ignore the extensive regulation already in place.

Based on the Council's public deliberations, over half of the Council do not have ethical problems with cloning-for-biomedical-research based simply on the status of the embryo. The proposal of a moratorium on SCNT, and not its outright ban, by the President's Council on Bioethics certainly implies that the Council deems this research to be important for medical science. A moratorium can only be counterproductive to the good that can come out of this research. Rather, the thoughtful application of current regulations to all SCNT research and consideration of independent efforts to regulate the market in human gametes will allow this research to proceed with its risks minimized and its benefits maximized for all.

ELIZABETH H. BLACKBURN

* * *

Statement of Professor Dresser

Below are my reasons for agreeing with the First Proposal.

I. Cloning to Have a Child

The ethical question presented today is not, "if cloning to have a child were safe, should it then be permitted?" Instead, the question is whether societies should allow scientists and physicians to conduct research aimed at producing babies through cloning. Posing the question this way highlights the research ethics issues raised by this form of cloning.

A central ethical issue is whether studies of cloning to have a child would present a balance of risks (to women, fetuses, children, and society) and expected benefits (to the child, prospective parents, and society) that justifies proceeding with human trials. The National Academy of Sciences (NAS) report *Scientific and Medical Aspects of Human Reproductive Cloning* observes that high numbers of human eggs would be required for this research. Women serving as research subjects would be exposed to the risks presented by fertility drugs and egg retrieval procedures. Women would also be exposed to risks associated with gestating a cloned fetus. As the NAS report notes, animals pregnant with cloned fetuses have had miscarriages and other health complications. If prenatal tests revealed problems in the fetus, women would face decisions about pregnancy termination. At least initially, human studies would expose children to the risk of disability and premature death. Parents and society could face burdens associated with caring for disabled children. Even if further cloning work in other species leads to better outcomes, good outcomes would not be assured in humans.

Added to these risks are the broader ethical concerns raised by cloning to have a child, such as psychological harm and objectification of children. Admittedly, many children today are born into environments that expose them to serious physical, social, and psychic harms. Prenatal and preimplantation screening allow parents to exercise deliberate control over children=s genetic makeup. Confused and difficult family relations can arise in "natural" family settings and as a result of currently practiced assisted reproduction methods. Certain social practices may allow and encourage parents to regard children as projects or products.

What is different about cloning is the array of risks and worries it presents, together with the relatively little that would be gained by developing the procedure. Although there are a few cases in which cloning to have a child might be morally acceptable, there are not enough of those cases to justify exposing research subjects and others to the harms that could accompany human testing.

Research on cloning to have children would also consume resources that might otherwise be devoted to more worthwhile projects. The limited resources available to support biomedical research should go to studies relevant to serious human health problems. Responsible companies and scientists ought to devote their efforts to research on important health problems, rather than on cloning to have children.

II. Cloning-for-Biomedical-Research

Several U.S. court opinions and advisory panel reports assign an intermediate moral status to the human embryo. According to these statements, embryos should be treated with special respect—not the respect we give to fully developed humans, but more respect than we give to items of property. One difficulty with the intermediate status position is that there is little clarity or agreement on what it means to treat human embryos with special respect.

Special respect might mean that embryos ought not be created purely for use as a research tool or a therapy to help others. Creating embryos for these purposes would represent a significant step beyond allowing the research use of donated IVF embryos that would otherwise be destroyed. Creating embryos for research would require women to provide eggs for research use. It is possible that payment would be necessary to attract a sufficient number of egg-providers (this would depend on the number of eggs needed and the number of women willing to donate for altruistic reasons). In this context, women would be helping to produce a research tool, rather than helping infertile people to have children.

Some people believe that creation of cloned and other embryos for research would be consistent with the special respect view. In 1994, a majority of the National Institutes of Health Human Embryo Research Panel said that creating embryos for research "for the most serious and compelling reasons" would be permissible. Former President Clinton disagreed with this judgment, however. And because panel Members themselves were concerned about the risks associated with egg donation, they recommended that eggs for research embryos be obtained solely from women already undergoing IVF for infertility treatment, women undergoing gynecological surgery for other reasons, and deceased women based on their previous consent or the consent of their next-of-kin. The deliberations in 1994 concerned acceptable conditions for government funding of human embryo research, but I do not think the participants meant to suggest that privately funded research should be evaluated according to wholly different moral considerations.

Because there are legitimate moral concerns raised by the practice of creating human embryos for research, I believe it would be premature to endorse cloning-for-biomedical-research. To approve cloning is to approve the creation of embryos as research tools. Past advisory groups and others have expressed sufficient reservations about this step to warrant more extensive national deliberation about whether it is justified at all and, if so, under what conditions.

I find it hard to reconcile the special respect view with a policy that allows embryos to be created purely as a research tool. I also recognize that some individuals assign a higher moral status to the early embryo. I do not want to endorse a practice that many people believe is wrong in the absence of compelling reasons to do so. At the same time, I can imagine studies that would offer sufficient benefit to patients to justify the creation of embryos for research through cloning or other methods.

For me, an important consideration is whether there are or will be in the near future alternative methods of investigating the relevant scientific questions. With regard to potential stem cell therapies, the question is whether cloning will be necessary to avoid the immune rejection problem. The NAS report *Stem Cells and the Future of Regenerative Medicine* repeatedly states that additional research in many areas is needed to determine whether embryonic stem cells can provide effective therapies to patients. A period of research focused on stem cells from donated embryos remaining after infertility treatment and on the immune rejection problem in animals could help to clarify whether it is necessary to move to research on stem cells from cloned human embryos. As for other types of research that might be conducted with stem cells from cloned human embryos, I believe scientists need to explain in more detail the significance of the research questions and the reasons why they cannot be investigated using alternative methods.

The appropriate oversight system is another matter meriting further analysis. In my view, proposals to create research embryos should be evaluated by a group that includes scientific experts, members of other professions, and ordinary citizens. The review group should include individuals with different positions on the moral status of early embryos. Approval should occur only after a rigorous and thorough analysis of individual proposals. The review group should require strong evidence that a proposal will generate information both relevant to a serious human health problem and not available through alternative research approaches.

I also believe that the temptation will be strong to extend the time limits for permissible human embryo and fetal research. Events in the past demonstrate that the desire to advance knowledge can lead to immoral research practices. Because there is likely to be pressure to allow destructive research on developing humans past the point at which stem cells can be retrieved, our nation should establish a strong moral and policy basis for drawing the line at a particular point in development.

In sum, I believe that a four-year moratorium on cloning-for-biomedical-research is justified for a variety of reasons. A moratorium gives scientists time to gather data and develop a stronger account of why it is necessary to obtain stem cells from cloned embryos. A moratorium allows Members of this Council and others to consider embryo cloning in its broader ethical and policy context and to deliberate about appropriate oversight structures for cloning and related practices. I hope that the moratorium also gives members of the public an opportunity to learn more about the actual state of stem cell research. This is truly a promising area, but it is far from certain that all or even some of its projected therapeutic benefits will materialize.

Finally, I hope that future public and policy discussions will confront the challenge of providing patients with access to any stem cell therapies that may be developed. Millions of patients in the United States lack access to established health care that could improve and extend their lives. People in developing countries lack access to the most basic medical assistance. Because helping patients is the ethical justification for conducting stem cell and other forms of biomedical research, improved access to existing and future therapies must be part of the national discussion.

REBECCA S. DRESSER

* * *

Statement of Dr. Foster

For Proposal Two

I begin by saying that the deliberations of the Council have been from the beginning serious, open and collegial. Although strong differences exist amongst some members, these have been expressed in scholarly and dignified fashion, without anger or personal attacks.

I support Proposal 2. The core issues in the discussion have been two. The first is "the nature of the embryo" argument. Some supporting Proposal 1 feel strongly that from the moment of conception, or the moment of cloning, the germ of potential life is so powerful as to render the nascent embryo deserving of protection equal to that of a full human. Others believe that respect for the embryo, though it is not yet fully human, requires a moratorium to see if alternatives might render cloning unnecessary. There is no doubt that a five or six day embryo is potentially human, but it cannot become a human by itself as would occur in normal human conception. The one or two hundred cell organism, the blastocyst, is neither viable nor feeling; there are no organs and there is no brain. There is nothing it can do without external help and implantation. From the standpoint of science it is potentially human but biologically pre-human. The evidence for this conclusion seems unarguable to me.

Proponents of Proposal 1, although they may agree with the biological facts, focus on "what might be" for the embryo. If implanted, some of the blastocysts from any source might become fully human, a child. However, in natural conception many embryos, perhaps half or more, are deleted in the first trimester. I calculated, using the World Health Organization 2001 estimate of about 360,000 births in the world each day, and assuming 50 percent implantation possibility, that more than 130 million embryos are lost naturally each year. Thus what any embryo might become is far from certain. Obviously the philosophical/moral argument of absolute or near absolute sanctity of any embryo cannot be answered by the scientific/biological argument. But I hold to the latter.

The "slippery slope" argument has been extensively discussed and fundamentally devolves to the fear or belief that lessons learned in cloning for research and therapy would make cloning-to-produce-children easier or more likely to occur. That is a legitimate fear, hence the desire by all of us for a ban on cloning-to-produce-children and the demand for regulation of all cloning.

I believe that biomedical science is a powerful good in the universe. The achievements in the prevention and cure of human disease and suffering over the past half century have been remarkable. What we know about nature grows daily. Stem cell research has great potential to take us further. Is it certain that dramatic health benefits will follow? Of course not. Science is a discipline of uncertainty. That is why in my view we should begin the research. I believe we have to compare the stem cells side by side: adult stem cells versus IVF stem cells versus cloned stem cells. Then we will know whether the potential is real and what the advantages or disadvantages of each cell type might be. Supporters of Proposal 1 also believe that research is necessary and argue that the moratorium will allow research on adult and IVF stem cells. But it eliminates a critical element, the direct comparison by controlled experiments for all three types of potentially therapeutic cells.

I said above that science is a discipline of uncertainty that requires experiments to answer questions of truth. It is also a discipline of hope. I believe that Proposal 2 is a very good thing for all those who suffer from disease. It is a decision for hope. It is for this reason that I support it.

DANIEL W. FOSTER

*   *   *

Statement of Dr. Gazzaniga

Oscar Wilde's lament, "A man who moralizes is usually a hypocrite," is a fairly rough statement. While I don't fully subscribe to it, I do believe that it cuts to the heart of much of the problematic nature of moralization: the divide that can exist between reasoning as reflected in actions in the face of a collection of facts and reasoning grounded on little more than a cultural belief system.

Of course, we are all free to have our views on everything from baseball to embryos. This is a large part of what makes this country great. But moralizers often go much further. Frequently, they want you to conform to their views, an agenda that I find entirely disturbing, and particularly troubling, when cast in the large, as a basis for social and even scientific policy.

My personal view on these matters is driven by forty years of scientific study on how the brain enables mind, which gives me a particular professional perspective on how our species forms and maintains its belief systems. This, for better or worse, is the lens through which I see these deliberations.

I disagree with most of the moral reasoning argued in this report. For me it is full of unsubstantiated psychological speculations on the nature of sexual life and theories of moral agency. In what follows, I state my position on the issue of both cloning-to-produce-children and cloning-for-biomedical-research in the form of a short essay. I try to capture my own passion for what is at stake.

Let Science Roll Forward

It was a bright and wintry January day when President Bush convened his advisory panel on bioethics in the Roosevelt Room of the White House. I was excited to be there and our charge was, and is, to see, explicate, and finally advise him how to respond to the flood of ethical complexities unearthed by the torrent of new biomedical technology. The President implored us to engage in that age-old technique of intellectual dueling that is debate. I was confident that a sensible and sensitive policy might evolve from what was sure to be a cacophony of voices of scientists and philosophers, representing a spectrum of opinions, beliefs, and intellectual backgrounds.

It was thus a surprise to me to hear the President's April speech on cloning. His opinions appeared fully formed, even though our panel had yet to finalize a report and still awaited a vote on the singularly crucial point of so-called cloning-for-biomedical-research. While it is true that the President's position is one held by some of the Members of the panel, it is not unanimous, and the panel's charge, the public nature of our panel's debate, and our national political process leave me wanting to make public my own personal view at this time.

Most people are aware that we no longer see cloning in a simple one-process-fits-all framework. At the very least there are two flavors. Cloning-to-produce-children is that process by which a new human being might be grown from the genetic material of a single individual. At this point in our history, no one supports cloning-to-produce-children. It is, by consensus, dangerous, probably not even attainable for years, and simply an odd concept. Even if cloning-to-produce-children did succeed in the future, the idea of informing one's spouse, "Let's go with my genes, not yours," is bizarre and socially a nonstarter.

In juxtaposition to cloning-to-produce-children is cloning-for-biomedical-research. This is another matter entirely. Cloning-for-biomedical-research is carried out with a completely different set of intentions from cloning-to-produce children. Cloning-for-biomedical-research is a bit of a misnomer, but it is the term the panel wants to use instead of "therapeutic cloning," for it is meant to cover not only cloning for therapeutics (for such diseases as diabetes, Parkinson's disease, and so on) but also that cloning now deemed necessary for understanding all genetic disorders. This is cloning for the sole purpose of enabling various types of lifesaving biomedical research. Perhaps the Council should have called it "lifesaving cloning."

Intentions aside, it is worth recalling the mechanics of cloning-for-biomedical-research. Scientists prefer to call this somatic cell nuclear transfer for a simple reason. That is all it is. Any cell from an adult can be placed in an egg whose own nucleus has been removed and given a jolt of electricity. This all takes place in a lab dish, and the hope is that this transfer will allow the adult cell to be reprogrammed so that it will form a clump of approximately 150 cells called a blastocyst. That clump of cells will then be harvested for the stem cells the clump contains, and medical science will move forward.

The general public gets confused around this point in a discussion. The confusions come from a conflation of ideas, beliefs, and facts. At the core seems to be the idea, asserted by some religious groups and some ethicists, that this moment of transfer of cellular material is an initiation of life, and so is the moment when a moral equivalency is established between a developing group of cells and a human being. They believe this is true for a normally sexually produced embryo and now so too for this new activated cell. This is the point of view that led to the President's view that both cloning-to-produce-children and cloning-for-biomedical-research should be outlawed. But in light of modern biological knowledge, is the view that life and moral agency start at the same time reasonable and true? Some think not.

First, consider embryos. We now know that as many as 50 to 80 percent of all fertilized eggs spontaneously abort. Those fertilized eggs are simply expelled from the body. It is hard to believe that under any religious belief system people would grieve and/or hold funerals for these natural events. Yet, if these unfortunate zygotes are considered human beings, then logically they should. Second, the process of a single zygote splitting to make identical twins can occur at least until fourteen days after fertilization. Thus, how could we possibly identify a person with a single fertilized egg? Additionally, even divided embryos can recombine back into one. The happy result would be a person who has emerged from two distinct fertilized eggs but is otherwise just like you and me. The "person = zygote" theory would have to say that he is two people! Finally, with respect to activated cells, there is no real claim when it all starts because it is not known in any detail.

Because the fertilization process is now understood, it serves as the modern scientific basis for the British position, which does not grant moral status to an embryo until after fourteen days, the time when all the twinning issues cease and the point where it must be implanted into the uterus if development is to continue. Thus, in Britain, embryo research goes on up to the blastocyst stage only and now, most recently, attempts at cloning to the blastocyst stage will be permitted.

The laboratory-devised blastocyst to be used for cloning-for-biomedical-research, the biological clump of cells at issue here, is the size of the dot on this "i." It has no nervous system and is therefore not sentient in any way and has no trajectory to becoming a human unless it is re-implanted into a women's uterus. And yet it likely carries the gold for the cure of millions of people. My brother is a general surgeon. He has saved hundreds of lives because he was able to transplant hearts and livers and kidneys and lungs to others from clinically brain-dead patients. The next of kin gave their loved one's tissue to help others, a practice which is condoned by all of society, including Catholics. It seems only right that those adults not needing leftover IVF embryos or eggs, neither of which have a brain at all, should have the same right to will them for use in biomedical research. The no-brained blastocyst that can develop from these tissue gifts, from both IVF and biomedical cloning technologies, is ready to help the suffering of brain-alive children and adults.

The President asked us to debate on our opening day. He said, "That's what I want. You haven't heard a debate until you have heard Colin Powell and Don Rumsfeld go at it." He lets these two trusted aides have it out, and I think he made a courageous and wise decision to send in the troops to have at the terrorists who would destroy innocent women and children. Disease does the same. I only hope he hears the debate, and then I hope he decides

to send in the stem cells to root out disease. In the spirit of these times, I too say, "Let's roll."

MICHAEL S. GAZZANIGA

∗   ∗   ∗

Statement of Professor George (Joined by Dr. Gómez-Lobo)

The subject matter of the present report is human cloning, the production of a human embryo by means of somatic cell nuclear transfer (SCNT) or similar technologies. Just as fertilization, if successful, generates a human embryo, cloning produces the same result by combining what is normally combined and activated in fertilization, that is, the full genetic code plus the ovular cytoplasm. Fertilization produces a new and complete, though immature, human organism. The same is true of successful cloning. Cloned embryos therefore ought to be treated as having the same moral status as other human embryos.

A human embryo is a whole living member of the species homo sapiens in the earliest stage of his or her natural development. Unless denied a suitable environment, an embryonic human being will by directing its own integral organic functioning develop himself or herself to the next more mature developmental stage, i.e., the fetal stage. The embryonic, fetal, infant, child, and adolescent stages are stages in the development of a determinate and enduring entity—a human being—who comes into existence as a single cell organism and develops, if all goes well, into adulthood many years later.*

Human embryos possess the epigenetic primordia for self-directed growth into adulthood, with their determinateness and identity fully intact. The adult human being that is now you or me is the same human being who, at an earlier stage of his or her life, was an adolescent, and before that a child, an infant, a fetus, and an embryo. Even in the embryonic stage, you and I were undeniably whole, living members of the species homo sapiens. We were then, as we are now, distinct and complete (though in the beginning we were, of course, immature) human organisms; we were not mere parts of other organisms.

Consider the case of ordinary sexual reproduction. Plainly, the gametes whose union brings into existence the embryo are not whole or distinct organisms. They are functionally (and not merely genetically) identifiable as *parts* of the male or female (potential) parents. Each has only half the genetic material needed to

---

* A human embryo (like a human being in the fetal, infant, child, or adolescent stage) is not properly classified as a "prehuman" organism with the mere potential to become a human being. No human embryologist or textbook in human embryology known to us presents, accepts, or remotely contemplates such a view. The testimony of all leading embryology textbooks is that a human embryo *is*—already and not merely potentially—a human being. His or her potential, assuming a sufficient measure of good health and a suitable environment, is to develop by an internally directed process of growth through the further stages of maturity on the continuum that is his or her life.

guide the development of an immature human being toward full maturity. They are destined either to combine with an oocyte or spermatozoon to generate a new and distinct organism, or simply die. Even when fertilization occurs, they do not survive; rather, their genetic material enters into the composition of a new organism.

But none of this is true of the human embryo, from the zygote and blastula stages onward. The combining of the chromosomes of the spermatozoon and of the oocyte generates what every authority in human embryology identifies as a new and distinct organism. Whether produced by fertilization or by SCNT or some other cloning technique, the human embryo possesses all of the genetic material needed to inform and organize its growth. Unless deprived of a suitable environment or prevented by accident or disease, the embryo is actively developing itself to full maturity. The direction of its growth *is not extrinsically determined,* but is in accord with the genetic information *within* it.* The human embryo is, then, a whole (though immature) and distinct human organism—a human being.

If the embryo were *not* a complete organism, then what could it be? Unlike the spermatozoa and the oocytes, it is not a part of the mother or of the father. Nor is it a disordered growth such as a hydatidiform mole or teratoma. (Such entities lack the internal resources to actively develop themselves to the next more mature stage of the life of a human being.) Perhaps someone will say that the early embryo is an intermediate form, something that regularly emerges into a whole (though immature) human organism but is not one yet. But what could cause the emergence of the whole human organism, and cause it with regularity? It is clear that from the zygote stage forward, the major development of this organism is *controlled and directed from within,* that is, by the organism itself. So, after the embryo comes into being, no event or series of events occur that could be construed as the production of a new organism; that is, nothing extrinsic to the developing organism itself acts on it to produce a new character or new direction in development.

But does this mean that the human embryo is a human being deserving of full moral respect such that it may not legitimately be used as a mere means to benefit others?

To deny that embryonic human beings deserve full respect, one must suppose that not every whole living human being is deserving of full respect. To do that, one must hold that those human beings who deserve full respect deserve it not in virtue of *the kind of entity they are,* but, rather, in virtue of some acquired characteristic that some human beings (or human beings at some stages) have and others

---

* The timing of the first two cleavages seems to be controlled by the maternal RNA within the embryo rather than by its new DNA (see Ronan O'Rahilly and Fabiola Mueller, *Human Embryology and Teratology* (New York: John Wiley & Sons, 1992), 23). Still, these cleavages do not occur if the embryo's nucleus is not present, and so the nuclear genes also control these early changes.

do not, and which some human beings have in greater degree than others.*

We submit that this position is untenable. It is clear that one need not be *actually* conscious, reasoning, deliberating, making choices, etc., in order to be a human being who deserves full moral respect, for it is clear that people who are asleep or in reversible comas deserve such respect. So, if one denied that human beings are intrinsically valuable in virtue of what they are, but required an additional attribute, the additional attribute would have to be a capacity of some sort, and, obviously a capacity for certain mental functions. Of course, human beings in the embryonic, fetal, and early infant stages lack immediately exercisable capacities for mental functions characteristically carried out (though intermittently) by most (not all—consider cases of severely retarded children and adults and comatose persons) human beings at later stages of maturity. Still, they possess in radical (= root) form these very capacities. Precisely by virtue of *the kind of entity they are,* they are from the beginning actively developing themselves to the stages at which these capacities will (if all goes well) be immediately exercisable. In this critical respect, they are quite unlike cats and dogs—even adult members of those species. As humans, they are members of a natural kind—the human species— whose embryonic, fetal, and infant members, if not prevented by some extrinsic cause, develop in due course and by intrinsic self-direction the immediately exercisable capacity for characteristically human mental functions. Each new human being comes into existence possessing the internal resources to develop immediately exercisable characteristically human mental capacities—and only the adverse effects on them *of other causes* will prevent their full development. In this sense, even human beings in the embryonic, fetal, and infant stages have the *basic natural* capacity for characteristically human mental functions.

---

* A possible alternative, though one finding little support in current discussions, would be to argue that what I am, or you are, is not a human organism at all, but rather a nonbodily consciousness or spirit merely inhabiting or somehow "associated with" a body. The problem with this argument is that it is clear that we *are* bodily entities—organisms, albeit of a particular type, namely, organisms of a rational nature. A living thing that performs bodily actions is an organism, a bodily entity. But it is immediately obvious in the case of the human individual that it is *the same subject* that perceives, walks, and talks (which are bodily actions), and that understands, deliberates, and makes choices—what everyone, including anyone who denies he is an organism, refers to as "I." It must be the same entity that perceives these words on a page, for example, and understands them. Thus, what each of us refers to as "I" is identically the physical organism that is the subject both of bodily actions, such as perceiving and walking, and of mental activities, such as understanding and choosing. Therefore, you and I are physical organisms, rather than consciousnesses that merely inhabit or are "associated with" physical organisms. And so, plainly, *we* came to be when the physical organism we are came to be; *we* once were embryos, then fetuses, then infants, and so on.

We can, therefore, distinguish two senses of the "capacity" (or what is sometimes referred to as the "potentiality") for mental functions: an immediately exercisable one, and a basic natural capacity, which develops over time. On what basis can one require for the recognition of full moral respect the first sort of capacity, which is an attribute that human beings acquire (if at all) only in the course of development (and may lose before dying), and that some will have in greater degree than others, and not the second, which is possessed by human beings as such? We can think of no good reason or nonarbitrary justification.

By contrast, there are good reasons to hold that the second type of capacity is the ground for full moral respect.

First, someone entertaining the view that one deserves full moral respect only if one has immediately exercisable capacities for mental functions should realize that the developing human being does not reach a level of maturity at which he or she performs a type of mental act that other animals do not perform—even animals such as dogs and cats—until at least several months after birth. A six-week-old baby lacks the *immediately exercisable* capacity to perform characteristically human mental functions. So, if full moral respect were due only to those who possess immediately exercisable capacities for characteristically human mental functions, it would follow that six-week-old infants do not deserve full moral respect. If one further takes the position that beings (including human beings) deserving less than full moral respect may legitimately be dismembered for the sake of research to benefit those who are thought to deserve full moral respect, then one is logically committed to the view that, subject to parental approval, the body parts of human infants, as well as those of human embryos and fetuses, should be fair game for scientific experimentation.

Second, the difference between these two types of capacity is merely a difference between stages along a continuum. The proximate, or immediately exercisable, capacity for mental functions is only the development of an underlying potentiality that the human being possesses simply by virtue of the kind of entity it is. The capacities for reasoning, deliberating, and making choices are gradually developed, or brought toward maturation, through gestation, childhood, adolescence, and so on. But the difference between a being that deserves full moral respect and a being that does not (and can therefore legitimately be dismembered as a means of benefiting others) cannot consist only in the fact that, while both have some feature, one has more of it than the other. A mere *quantitative* difference (having more or less of the same feature, such as the development of a basic natural capacity) cannot by itself be a justificatory basis for treating different entities in *radically* different ways. Between the ovum and the approaching thousands of sperm, on the one hand, and the embryonic human being, on the other hand, there *is* a clear difference in kind. But between the embryonic human being and that same human being at any later stage of its maturation, there is only a difference in degree.

Third, being a whole human organism (whether immature or not) is an either/or matter—a thing either is or is not a whole human being. But the acquired qualities that could be proposed as criteria for personhood come in varying and continuous degrees: there is an infinite number of degrees of the relevant developed abilities or dispositions, such as for self-consciousness, intelligence, or rationality. So, if human beings were worthy of full moral respect only because of such qualities, and not in virtue of the kind of being they are, then, since such qualities come in varying degrees, no account could be given of why basic rights are not possessed by human beings in varying degrees. The proposition that all human beings are created equal would be relegated to the status of a superstition. For example, if developed self-consciousness bestowed rights, then, since some people are more self-conscious than others (that is, have developed that capacity to a greater extent than others), some people would be greater in dignity than others, and the rights of the superiors would trump those of the inferiors where the interests of the superiors could be advanced at the cost of the inferiors. This conclusion would follow no matter which of the acquired qualities generally proposed as qualifying some human beings (or human beings at some stages) for full respect were selected. Clearly, developed self-consciousness, or desires, or so on, are arbitrarily selected degrees of development of capacities that all human beings possess in (at least) radical form from the coming into being of the organism until his or her death. So, it cannot be the case that *some* human beings *and not others* are intrinsically valuable, by virtue of a certain degree of development. Rather, human beings are intrinsically valuable *in virtue of what (i.e., the kind of being) they are*; and *all* human beings—not just some, and certainly not just those who have advanced sufficiently along the developmental path as to be able to exercise their capacities for characteristically human mental functions—are intrinsically valuable.

Since human beings are intrinsically valuable and deserving of full moral respect in virtue of what they are, it follows that they are intrinsically valuable from the point at which they come into being. Even in the embryonic stage of our lives, each of us was a human being and, as such, worthy of concern and protection. Embryonic human beings, whether brought into existence by union of gametes, SCNT, or other cloning technologies, should be accorded the status of inviolability recognized for human beings in other developmental stages.

Three arguments have been repeatedly advanced in the course of our Council's deliberations in an effort to cast doubt on the proposition that human embryos deserve to be accorded such status.

(1) Some have claimed that the phenomenon of monozygotic twinning shows that the embryo in the first several days of its gestation is not a human individual. The suggestion is that as long as twinning can occur, what exists is not yet a unitary human being but only a mass of cells—each cell is totipotent and allegedly independent of the others.

It is true that *if a cell or group of cells is detached from the whole* at an early stage of embryonic development, then what is detached can sometimes become a distinct organism and has the potential to develop to maturity as distinct from the embryo from which it was detached (this is the meaning of "totipotent"). But this does nothing to show that before detachment the cells within the human embryo constituted only an incidental mass. Consider the parallel case of division of a flatworm. Parts of a flatworm have the potential to become a whole flatworm when isolated from the present whole of which they are part. Yet no one would suggest that prior to the division of a flatworm to produce two whole flatworms the original flatworm was not a unitary individual. Likewise, at the early stages of human embryonic development, before specialization by the cells has progressed very far, the cells or groups of cells can become whole organisms if they are divided and have an appropriate environment after the division. But that fact does not in the least indicate that prior to such an extrinsic division the embryo is other than a unitary, self-integrating, actively developing human organism. It certainly does not show that the embryo is a mere clump of cells.

In the first two weeks, the cells of the developing embryonic human being already manifest a degree of specialization or differentiation. From the very beginning, even at the two-cell stage, the cells differ in the cytoplasm received from the original ovum. Also they are differentiated by their position within the embryo. In mammals, even in the unfertilized ovum, there is already an "animal" pole (from which the nervous system and eyes develop) and a "vegetal" pole (from which the future "lower" organs and the gut develop).[*] After the initial cleavage, the cell coming from the "animal" pole is probably the primordium of the nervous system and the other senses, and the cell coming from the "vegetal" pole is probably the primordium of the digestive system. Moreover, the relative position of a cell from the very beginning (that is, from the first cleavage) has an impact on its functioning. Monozygotic twinning usually occurs at the blastocyst stage, in which there clearly is a differentiation of the inner cell mass and the trophoblast that surrounds it (from which the placenta develops).[†]

The orientation and timing of the cleavages are species specific, and are therefore genetically determined, that is, determined from within. Even at the two-cell stage, the embryo begins synthesizing a glycoprotein called "E-cadherin" or "uvomorulin," which will be instrumental in the compaction process at the eight-cell stage, the process in which the blastomeres (individual cells of the embryo at the blastocyst stage) join tightly together, flattening and developing an inside-outside polarity.[‡] And there is still more evidence, but the point is that from the

---

Werner A. Muller, *Developmental Biology* (New York: Springer Verlag, 1997), 12 f. Scott Gilbert, *Developmental Biology* 5th edition (Sunderland, Mass.: Sinnauer Associates, 1997); O'Rahilly and Mueller, *Human Embryology and Teratology*, 23-24.

[†] O'Rahilly and Fabiola Mueller, *Human Embryology and Teratology*, 30-31.

[‡] Ibid. 23-24; Keith Moore, and T.V.N. Persaud, *Before We Are Born: Essentials of Embryology and Birth Defects* (Philadelphia: W.B. Saunders, 1998), 41; William J.

zygote stage forward, the embryo, as well as maintaining homeostasis, is internally integrating various processes to direct them in an overall growth pattern toward maturity.*

But the clearest evidence that the embryo in the first two weeks is not a mere mass of cells but is a unitary organism is this: *if the individual cells within the embryo before twinning were each independent of the others, there would be no reason why each would not regularly develop on its own. Instead, these allegedly independent, noncommunicating cells regularly function together to develop into a single, more mature member of the human species.* This fact shows that interaction is taking place between the cells from the very beginning (even within the zona pellucida, before implantation), restraining them from individually developing as whole organisms and directing each of them to function as a relevant part of a single, whole organism continuous with the zygote. Thus, prior to an extrinsic division of the cells of the embryo, these cells together do constitute a single organism. So, the fact of twinning does not show that the embryo is a mere incidental mass of cells. Rather, the evidence clearly indicates that the human embryo, from the zygote stage forward, is a unitary, human organism.

(2) The second argument we wish to address suggests that since people frequently do not grieve, or do not grieve intensely, for the loss of an embryo early in pregnancy, as they do for the loss of a fetus late in pregnancy or of a newborn, we are warranted in concluding that the early embryo is not a human being worthy of full moral respect.

The absence of grieving is sometimes a result of ignorance about the facts of embryogenesis and intrauterine human development. If people are told (as they still are in some places) that there simply is no human being until "quickening"— a view which is preposterous in light of the embryological facts—then they are likely not to grieve (or not to grieve intensely) at an early miscarriage. But people who are better informed, and women in particular, very often *do* grieve even when a miscarriage occurs early in pregnancy.

Granted, some people informed about many of the embryological facts are nevertheless indifferent to early miscarriages; but this is often due to a reductionist view according to which embryonic human beings are misdescribed as mere "clumps of cells," "masses of tissue," etc. The *emotional* attitude one has toward early miscarriages is typically and for the most part *an effect* of what one thinks— rightly or wrongly—about the humanity of the embryo. Hence it is circular reasoning to use the indifference of people who deny (wrongly, in our view) that human beings in the embryonic stage deserve full moral respect as an argument

---

Larson, *Human Embryology* 3rd edition (New York: Churchill Livingstone, 2001), 18-21.

* Gilbert, *Developmental Biology*, 12 f; 167 f. Also see O'Rahilly and Mueller, *Human Embryology and Teratology* 23-24.

for not according such respect.

Moreover, the fact that people typically grieve less in the case of a miscarriage than they do in the case of an infant's death is partly explained by the simple facts that they do not actually see the baby, hold her in their arms, talk to her, and so on. The process of emotional bonding is typically completed after the child is born—sometimes, and in some cultures, months after the child is born. However, a child's right not to be killed plainly does not depend on whether her parents or anyone else has formed an emotional bond with her. Every year—perhaps every day—people die for whom others do not grieve. This does not mean that they lacked the status of human beings who were worthy of full moral respect.

It is simply a mistake to conclude from the fact that people do not grieve, or grieve less, at early miscarriage that the embryo has in herself less dignity or worth than older human beings.

(3) We now turn to the third argument. Some people, apparently, are moved to believe that embryonic human beings are not worthy of full moral respect because a high percentage of embryos formed in natural pregnancies fail to implant or spontaneously abort. Again, we submit that the inference is fallacious.

It is worth noting first, as the standard embryology texts point out, that many of these unsuccessful pregnancies are really due to incomplete fertilizations. So, in many cases, what is lost is not actually a human embryo. To be a complete human organism (a human being), the entity must have the epigenetic primordia for a functioning brain and nervous system, though a chromosomal defect might only prevent development to maximum functioning (in which case it would be a human being, though handicapped). If fertilization is not complete, then what is developing is not an organism with the active capacity to develop itself to the mature (even if handicapped) state of a human.

Second, the argument here rests upon a variant of the naturalistic fallacy. It supposes that what happens in "nature," i.e., with predictable frequency without the intervention of human agency, must be morally acceptable when deliberately caused. Since embryonic death in early miscarriages happens with predictable frequency without the intervention of human agency, the argument goes, we are warranted in concluding that the deliberate destruction of human beings in the embryonic stage is morally acceptable.

The unsoundness of such reasoning can easily be brought into focus by considering the fact that historically, and in some places even today, the *infant* mortality rate has been very high. If the reasoning under review here were sound, it would show that human infants in such circumstances could not be full human beings possessing a basic right not to be killed for the benefit of others. But that of course is surely wrong. The argument is a *non sequitur*.

In conclusion, we submit that law and public policy should proceed on the basis of full moral respect for human beings irrespective of age, size, stage of development, or condition of dependency. Justice requires no less. In the context of the debate over cloning, it requires, in our opinion, a ban on the production of embryos, whether by SCNT or other processes, for research that harms them or results in their destruction. Embryonic human beings, no less than human beings at other developmental stages, should be treated as subjects of moral respect and human rights, not as objects that may be damaged or destroyed for the benefit of others. We also hold that cloning-to-produce-children ought to be legally prohibited. In our view, such cloning, even if it could be done without the risk of defects or deformities, treats the child-to-be as a product of manufacture, and is therefore inconsistent with a due respect for the dignity of human beings. Still, it is our considered judgment that cloning-for-biomedical-research, inasmuch as it involves the deliberate destruction of embryos, is morally worse than cloning-to-produce-children. Thus we urge that any ban on cloning-to-produce-children be a prohibition on the practice of cloning itself, and not on the implantation of embryos. Public policy should protect embryonic human beings and certainly not mandate or encourage their destruction. An effective ban on cloning-to-produce-children would be a ban on all cloning.[*]

Although an optimal policy would permanently ban all cloning, we join in this Council's call for a permanent ban on cloning-to-produce-children combined with a four-year ban (or "moratorium") on cloning-for-biomedical-research for the reasons set forth by Gilbert Meilaender in his personal statement. It is our particular hope that a four-year period will provide time for a careful and thorough public debate about the moral status of the human embryo. This is a debate we welcome.

ROBERT P. GEORGE
ALFONSO GÓMEZ-LOBO

* * *

[*] A ban on implantation of an existing embryo or class of embryos would be subject to constitutional as well as moral objections. Such a ban would certainly be challenged, and the challenge would likely come from a powerful coalition of "pro-life" and "pro-choice" forces. A prohibition of the production of embryos by cloning would have a far better likelihood of withstanding constitutional challenge than would a ban on implantation.

Statement of Dr. Hurlbut

In joining with fellow Members of the Council in support of a moratorium on cloning for biomedical research, I consider this recommendation not an admission of ambivalence on matters of policy, but a recognition of the difficulty of the moral issues involved and an affirmation of the need for further discussion and deliberation. Throughout our proceedings it has become increasingly apparent that without clear and distinct moral principles, grounded in scientific evidence and reasoned moral argument, no policy can be effectively formulated or enforced. Most specifically, the proposed limitation of fourteen days for research on human embryos and the prohibition against implantation appear to be arbitrarily set and therefore vulnerable to transgression through the persuasive promise of further scientific benefit. Clearly, a more thorough and thoughtful consideration of the moral status of the human embryo is warranted. It is in the spirit of this continuing discussion that I offer the personal perspectives that follow.

Introduction

In pondering the ethics of cloning-for-biomedical-research it is apparent that as our science is changing, so is the nature of our moral dilemmas. Each advance forces us to think more deeply about what it means to be human. As the scientific focus on genomics moves on to proteomics and now to the early stages of the study of developmental biology, we are confronted with the challenge of understanding the moral meaning of human life in its dynamics of change, as both potential and process.

A reasonable anticipation of the likely course of science suggests that concerns about cloning are just the beginning of a series of difficult ethical issues relating to embryo experimentation and medical intervention in developing life. In addition, advances in developmental biology will open more deeply the dilemmas related to human-animal hybridization, extra-corporeal gestation, and genetic and cellular enhancement. Driven by the vast range of research applications and opportunities for clinical interventions in disease and disability (especially the open ended possibilities promised by regenerative medicine) this technology will be powerfully propelled into the forefront of medical science.

Given the complex course of science and the drive to its development, any moral assessment of cloning-for-biomedical-research (CBR) must describe the central human goods it seeks to preserve, the range and boundaries of these values, and the broad implications for science and society implied by them. Such an assessment should serve the dual purpose of helping to define the moral dangers while clearing the course for the fullest and most open future for scientific investigation and application.

Moral Principles

Although there are already numerous promising approaches for research on human development even without cloning-for-biomedical-research (CBR), I believe this technology could provide valuable tools for scientific inquiry and medical advance. In my judgment, the moral imperative to foster an increase of knowledge and new modes of therapeutic intervention weighs heavily in the equation of consideration. Nonetheless, I believe that, as they stand, current proposals for CBR will breach fundamental moral goods, erode social cohesion and ultimately constrain the promise of advances in developmental biology and their medical applications. However, there may be morally acceptable ways of employing CBR that could both preserve our commitment to fundamental moral principles and strengthen our appreciation of the significance of developing life, while also opening avenues of advance less limiting and more promising than the current scientific proposals.

The principle of human life as the fundamental good serves as the cornerstone of law for our civilization. In no circumstance is the intentional destruction of the life of an innocent individual deemed morally acceptable. Even where a right to abortion is given, for example, it is based on a woman's right not to be encumbered, a right of privacy, not a right to directly kill the fetus.* This valuing of human life is indeed the moral starting point for both advocates and opponents of CBR. This principle of the inviolability of human life is the reciprocal respect that we naturally grant as we recognize in the other a being of moral equivalence to ourselves. Although different cultures and different eras have affirmed this recognition in varied ways, I will argue that it is reasonable in light of our current scientific knowledge that we extend this principle to human life in its earliest developmental stages.

Life as Process

When looked at through the lens of science, it is evident that human existence cannot be defined atemporally, but must be recognized in the full procession of continuity and change that is essential for its development. From conception, our unique genetic endowment organizes and guides the expression of our particular nature in its species and individual character. Fertilization initiates the most complex chemical reaction in the known universe: a self-directing, purposeful integration of organismal development. In both character and conduct the zygote and subsequent embryonic stages differ from any other cells or tissues of the body; they contain within themselves the organizing principle of the full human organism.

This is not an abstract or hypothetical potential in the sense of mere possibility,

---

* If the fetus is delivered alive during an abortion, there is a legal obligation to resuscitate and sustain its life.

but rather a potency, an engaged and effective potential-in-process, an activated dynamic of development in the direction of human fullness of being. For this reason a zygote (or a clonote) differs fundamentally from an unfertilized egg, a sperm cell, or later somatic cells; it possesses an inherent organismal unity and potency that such other cells lack. Unlike an assembly of parts in which a manufactured product is in no sense "present" until there is a completed construction, a living being has a continuous unfolding existence that is inseparable from its emerging form. The form is itself a dynamic process rather than a static structure. In biology, the whole (as the unified organismal principle of growth) precedes and produces the parts. It is this implicit whole, with its inherent potency, that endows the embryo with its human character and therefore its inviolable moral status. To interfere in its development is to transgress upon a life in process.[*]

The argument is sometimes made that potential should not be part of the moral equation because of the low probability of successful development of the early embryo.[†] This, however, is itself an argument based on potential, in this case the lack of potential to develop normally.[‡] The fact that life in its early stages is extremely fragile and often fails is not an argument to lessen the moral standing of the embryo. Vulnerability does not render a life less valuable.

Accrued Moral Status

The major alternative to the view that an embryo has an inherent moral status is the assertion that moral status is an accrued or accumulated quality related to

---

[*] To recognize a potential as in some sense "actual" and worthy of protection, we need only consider how we would react to the intentional sterilization of a prepubescent girl when her fertility was only potential yet precious to her larger dignity and developmental integrity as a human person.

[†] Such an argument might hold some weight if one could argue that a given stage of development represents an emergent state in which a relational property is in ontological discontinuity with the material from which it emerged. At first consideration, this seems true of all biological systems where the whole reveals properties unpredicted within the parts. The problem in this line of reasoning, however, is that these properties are exactly that to which the whole is ordered and so are inherent powers, "actual" within the whole when seen across time. To know what a biological being is, we must observe it over time, understand it across its life span. It is the essence of life that it is ordered to employ these *leaps to* emergent states as an agency in development. New realities will emerge; this is established in the potency of the developing organism.

[‡] A similar problem arises in clinical medicine. It is crucial that we not equate the statistical probability of a specific outcome with the actual prognosis of the individual patient involved.

some dimension of form or function. Several arguments have been put forward for this position.

1. Gastrulation

One such accrual argument is based on the idea that before gastrulation (designated as the fourteenth day) the embryo is an inchoate clump of cells with no actuated drive in the direction of distinct development.* It is argued that the undifferentiated quality of the blastocyst justifies its disaggregation for the procurement of stem cells, while the evident organization at gastrulation reveals an organismal integrity that endows inviolable moral status to all subsequent stages of embryological development. Scientific evidence, however, supports the argument that from conception there is an unbroken continuity in the differentiation and organization of the emerging individual life. The anterior-posterior axis appears to be already established within the zygote, early cell divisions (at least after the eight-cell stage) exhibit differential gene expression† and unequal cytoplasmic concentrations of cell constituents suggest distinct cellular fates. This implies that the changes at gastrulation do not represent a discontinuity of ontological significance, but merely the visibly evident culmination of more subtle developmental processes (at the cellular level) driving in the direction of organismal maturity.

---

* The differentiation of the trophoblast, which will form the extra-embryonic membranes, is generally considered as distinct from the embryo itself. More true to the nature of life, it might be recognized as an organ of embryogenesis used and discarded within the dynamic process of development. Throughout the continuum of human life, from the embryo to the adult, cells, tissues and organs are reabsorbed, transcended and transformed. Examples include the umbilical vein and arteries (which become supporting ligaments), neurologic cells (more than half of which are culled by apoptosis and reabsorption), systems of reflexes (such as the moro reflex which is manifest only in infants), immune organs and functions such as the thymus (which shrivels in an adult), and allergies (which change throughout life and generally wane in mid-life). We do not just develop and then age, but undergo a continuous transformation and fuller manifestation of our organismal nature present within the earliest embryo.

† In fact, the first several cell divisions after natural fertilization do not require a nucleus to be present and therefore may not involve gene expression from the newly united bi-parental genetic material. The mRNA essential for protein synthesis at these early stages appears to be generated during the maturation of the egg and then remains dormant until after fertilization. This may very well preclude the possibilities of the optimistic but simplistic proposal that merely by adding a recipe of cytoplasmic factors essential for reprogramming we could transform any cell into a functional zygote. Nonetheless, even without differential gene expression, cytoplasmic studies reveal unequal cytoplasmic distributions, and implicit differential cell fates, even at these early stages.

2. Twinning

Another argument for accrued moral status is that as long as an embryo is capable of giving rise to a twin it cannot be considered to have the moral standing of an individual. There is the obvious objection that as one locus of moral status becomes two it does not diminish but increases the moral moment. But perhaps more substantially, this argument actually supports the notion that crucial dimensions of individuation (and their disruption that results in twinning) are already at work in the blastocyst, the stage at which most twinning occurs. Monozygotic twinning (a mere 0.4 percent of births) does not appear to be either an intrinsic drive or a random process within embryogenesis. Rather, it is a disruption of normal development by a mechanical or biochemical disturbance of fragile cell relationships that provokes a compensatory repair, but with the restitution of integrity within two distinct trajectories of embryological development.* In considering the implications of twinning for individuation, one might ask the question from the opposite perspective. What keeps each of these totipotent cells from becoming a full embryo? Clearly, crucial relational dynamics of position and intercellular communication are already at work establishing the unified pattern of the emerging individual. From this perspective twinning is not evidence of the absence of an individual, but of an extraordinary power of compensatory repair that reflects more fully the potency of the individual drive to fullness of form.

3. Implantation

Some have argued that the implantation of the embryo within the uterine lining of the mother constitutes a moment of altered moral status. Implantation, however, is actually a process that extends from around the sixth or seventh day to about the eleventh or twelfth day when the uteroplacental circulation is established. This complex circulatory exchange extends the earlier relationship between mother and embryo in which physiological conditions, including the diffusion of essential nutrients, sustained the life and nourished the growth of the developing embryo. Although these early conditions can be artificially simulated as in IVF, the delicate balance of essential factors and their effect on development (as seen in Large Offspring Syndrome)† is evidence of the crucial contribution of

---

* The fact that these early cells retain the ability to form a second embryo is testimony to the resiliency of self-regulation and compensation within early life, not the lack of individuation of the first embryo from which the second can be considered to have "budded" off. Evidence for this may be seen in the increased incidence of monozygotic twinning associated with IVF by Blastocyst Transfer. When IVF embryos are transferred to the uterus for implantation at the blastocyst stage, there is a two to ten-fold increase in the rate of monozygotic twinning, apparently due to disruption of normal organismal integrity. It is also interesting to note that with Blastocyst Transfer there is a slightly higher rate of male births.

† In some animal studies, it has been noted that particular components in the culture medium in which the embryo is nourished increase the size of the off-

the mother even in the first week of embryogenesis. Changes in the intricate interrelations between mother and infant cannot be viewed as an alteration of moral status, but as part of the ongoing epigenetic process all along the continuum of natural development that begins with conception and continues into infancy. This continuity implies no meaningful moral marker at implantation.[*]

4. Function

Arguments for a change in moral status based on function are at once the most difficult to refute and to defend. The first and most obvious problem is that the essential functions (even their minimal criteria and age of onset) are diverse and arbitrarily assigned. Generally they relate to the onset of sentience, awareness of pain, or some apparently unique human cognitive capability such as consciousness.[†] But if human moral worth is based on actual manifest functions, then does more of a particular function give an individual life a higher moral value? And what are we to make of the parallel capacities in animals that we routinely sacrifice for food and medical research? Furthermore, what becomes of human moral status with the degeneration or disappearance of such a function? While we might argue that our relational obligations change along with changes in function, such as occur with senile dementia, we would not sanction a utilitarian calculus and the purely instrumental use of such persons no matter how promising the medical benefits might be. The diagnostic requirements of "brain death" for removing organs for transplantation, far from being a justification for interrupting a developing life before "brain birth", actually point to the moral significance of potential and the stringency of the criteria for irreversible disintegration and death.

From a scientific perspective, there is no meaningful moment when one can definitively designate the biological origins of a human characteristic such as consciousness. Even designations such as 'the nervous system' are conceptual tools, reifications of an indivisible organismal unity. Zygote, morula, embryo, fetus, child and adult: these are conceptual constructions for convenience of descrip-

---

spring during later stages of gestation.

[*] It should be noted that this argument could be used as a counter-argument against the disaggregation of the preimplantation embryo, or as a justification for the production of more advanced cells, tissues, and organs either through implantation into an artificial endometrium or through natural gestation.

[†] In fact, from a scientific perspective, we should have a measure of humility when drawing conclusions about moral status from evidence concerning consciousness or capacities involving subjective experience. The fact that consciousness and subjective awareness appear to be mediated by matter does not exhaust their mystery.

tion, not distinct ontological categories. With respect to fundamental moral status therefore, as distinguished from developing relational obligations, the human being is an embodied being whose intrinsic dignity is inseparable from its full procession of life and always present in its varied stages of emergence.

A Bright Line at Conception

If the embryo has an inherent moral status that is not an accrued or accumulated quality related to some dimension of form or function, then that moral status must begin with the zygote (or clonote). Anything short of affirming the inviolability of life across all of its stages from zygote to natural death leads to an instrumental view of human life. Such a revocation of our most fundamental moral principle would reverse a long and overarching trend of progress in moral awareness and practice in our civilization. From human sacrifice,* to slavery, child labor, women's rights and civil rights, we have progressively discerned and prohibited practices that subject the individual to the injustice of exploitation by others. The reversal of such a basic moral valuation will extend itself in a logic of justification that has ominous implications for our attitude and approach to human existence. This is not a mere "slippery slope," where we are slowly led downward by the ever more desirable extension of exceptions to moral principle. It is, rather, a "crumbly cliff" where the very utility of abrogating a basic moral prohibition carries such convenience of consequence that the subsequent descent is simply practice catching up with principle.

The inviolability of human life is the essential foundation on which all other principles of justice are built, and any erosion of this foundation destabilizes the social cooperation that makes possible the benefits of organized society. Medicine is especially vulnerable to such effects since it operates at the intrinsically moral interface between scientific technique and the most tender and sensitive dimensions of personal reality in the vulnerable patient. As we descend into an instrumental use of human life we destroy the very reason for which we were undertaking our new therapies; we destroy the humanity we were trying to heal.

The promise of stem cells lies beyond simple cell cultures and cell replacement therapies. The fourteen-day marker will not hold up to logical argument.† The

---

* The sacrifice of infants for the supposed larger flourishing of life bespeaks the potency ascribed to purity and generative potential.

† The designation of fourteen days as the moral boundary for embryo experimentation is in the category of a "received tradition," almost a superstition in the sense that it is a belief in a change of state without a discernible cause. The validity of this designated moral marker has not been reexamined in the light of recent advances in our understanding of developmental biology. As a moral marker of ontological change fourteen days makes no sense. Even if one disagrees with the discussion above, the date should be set earlier: implantation is complete by the twelfth day, the onset of gastrulation occurs between the twelfth and fourteenth

technological goal is to produce the more advanced cell types of tissues, organs, and possibly even limb primordia. Producing such complex tissues and organs may require the cell interactions and microenvironments now available only through natural gestation.* The benefits of implanting cloned embryos (either into the natural womb or possibly an artificial endometrium) so as to employ the developmental dynamics of natural embryogenesis seem self-evident. The implantation of cloned embryos for the production of patient-specific tissue types to bypass problems of immune rejection would further extend the logic of the instrumental use of developing life. The public pressure that has already been brought to bear on the politics of stem cells and cloning by patient advocacy groups has provoked such a sense of promise that it may propel the argument for allowing implantation of cloned embryos. Different people may have different limits to the duration of gestation they find morally acceptable, but in light of the current sanction of abortion up to and beyond the end of the second trimester, it is difficult to argue that creation, gestation and sacrifice of a clone to save an existing life is a large leap in the logic of justification.

A Speculative Proposal

While maintaining a bright line at conception safeguards our most fundamental moral principle, the challenge remains to find an acceptable method of drawing on the great medical promise of CBR while precluding its use in ways that degrade the dignity of human existence. Some proponents of CBR maintain that the laboratory creation of the cloned embryo makes it a "pseudo-embryo" or "artifact," a product of human technological production.† The problem with this assertion is that, once created, the cloned embryo appears to be no different than

---

day and twinning is rare after the ninth day. Furthermore, it is worth noting that fourteen days is not of current scientific relevance since stem cells can be procured at the four-five day stage and, with present technology, human embryos can sustain viability in culture for only eight-nine days.

* Natural development proceeds within the context of a highly refined spatial and temporal niche of organized complexity of positional cues, signal diffusion and cell-cell contact between cellular lineages of diverse types. See for example the recent article, "Dominant role of the niche in melanocyte stem-cell fate determination" (*Nature* 25 April 2002).

† In fact, there will be several (and perhaps numerous) ways to produce cloned blastocysts from which stem cells can be harvested. These include: the current common method of cloning designated somatic cell nuclear transfer (SCNT) or nuclear transplantation, embryo splitting, use of animal oocytes as receptacles of nuclear transfer, fusion of embryonic stem cells and possibly fetal or adult stem cells into existing blastocysts and possibly the production of artificial gametes for the transfer of adult nuclear material, (and probably others more difficult to anticipate or legally regulate).

the product of natural fertilization. But what if we could use the cloning techniques of nuclear transfer to create an entity that lacks the qualities and capabilities essential to be designated a human life in process? By intentional alteration of the somatic cell nuclear components or the cytoplasm of the oocyte into which they are transferred, could we truly create an artifact (a human creation for human ends) that is biologically and morally more akin to tissue or cell culture?*

The intention in creating such an intrinsically limited "clonal artifact" would not be one of reproduction, but simply the desire to draw on natural organic potential through technological manipulation of biological materials. This intention is in keeping with the purposes of scientific research and medical therapy in which many "unnatural" manipulations are used for human benefit. In order to employ such an entity for research, it must be capable of yielding stem cells while lacking the capacity for the self-directed, integrated organic functioning that is essential for embryogenesis. The intervention that precludes the possibility of human development would be undertaken at a stage before the development was initiated, and thus, no active potentiality, no human life in process, would be violated. If the created artifact were accorded a certain cautionary respect (as with all human tissues), even though not the full protection of human life, the consequences of such a program would not compromise any moral principle.

The project of creating these altered "clonal artifacts" for the procurement of human stem cells could have many loci of scientific intervention. Techniques might range from removing genes for extra-embryonic structures, to the alteration of genes for angiogenesis (such that the stem cells procured could produce differentiated cell types with therapeutic potential, but would have to rely on the host into whom they were placed for their vascular connections). If the created stem cells could only form specific germ layers or limited lineages of cell types, they still might be useful for the generation of valuable research models as well as many cell lines, tissues and organs. Furthermore, in bypassing the moral concerns associated with full embryonic potential, the created cells might legitimately be developed within artificial microenvironments beyond fourteen days. This would allow the production of more advanced cell types, the study of tissue interactions and the formation of primordial organismal parts. Just as we have learned that neither genes, nor cells, nor even whole organs define the locus of human moral standing, in this era of developmental biology we will come to recognize that tissues with "partial generative potential" may be used for medical benefit without a violation of human dignity.† The fact that one does not need full embryonic in-

---

* Such a procedure could be designated "Altered Nuclear Transfer" (ANT).

† Consider blood transfusions, organ transplantation, and the recombination of human genes into bacteria for the production of human hormones such as growth hormone and insulin. All of these raised initial moral controversy until it was recognized that the locus of human dignity lies not it human parts but in the full organismal integrity of a human life.

tegrity for these partial generative capacities is evident in the well-formed body parts such as teeth, fingernails and hair seen in teratomas.*

Clearly, there will be some point where partial generative potential is so close to full human development that our basic moral principals would be violated. We will need to carefully define the circumstances under which it is acceptable for serious medical purposes to manipulate human parts apart from their natural context in human development. Here the fundamental principle of protection of human life must be affirmed, while the more subtle moral issues concerning respect and natural integrity are carefully explored.

At this early stage in our technological control of developing life, we have an opportunity to break the impasse over stem cell research and provide moral guidance for the biotechnology of the future. This may require a constructive reformulation of some aspects of moral philosophy, together with creative exploration of scientific possibilities, but any postponement of this process will only deepen the dilemma as we proceed into realms of technological advance unguided by forethought. A moratorium will allow the cooperative dialogue that is essential to frame the moral principles that can at once defend human dignity and promote the fullest prospects for scientific progress and its medical applications.

WILLIAM B. HURLBUT

*   *   *

---

*These benign ovarian tumors, derived by spontaneous and disorganized development of activated ova, typically have a full array of primary tissue types and some well-developed body parts. The possibility that embryonic stem cells could be derived from entities lacking integrated developmental potential is given further support from recent studies in which cells from abnormal early embryos were fused with normal embryos and went on to produce normal tissues in the developed organism. (See "Dependable Cells From Defective Embryos." *Science* 3 May 2002, p. 841, and Byrne, Simons and Gurdon: *Proceedings of the National Academy of Sciences (PNAS)* online, April 23, 2002.)

Statement of Dr. Krauthammer

I oppose all cloning, reproductive and research. I would like to see them banned. But I live in the real world. As I have explained, both in the Council and in my writings, I oppose research cloning for prudential reasons. Prudence dictates taking into account the real world, meaning the realities of American democracy, and at present there is no consensus for banning research cloning. I therefore strongly support a moratorium. At this point in the history of this debate, a moratorium is more than a compromise. It is an important achievement.

Let's remember. In a democracy, there is no such thing as a permanent ban in any case. Any ban can be revisited at any time. Thus the difference between a ban and a moratorium is simply this: Under a ban, when the issue is reconsidered, the burden of proof is on those who wish to lift the ban. With a moratorium, when the issue is reconsidered, the burden of proof is on those who wish to maintain the ban. I have no trepidation about remaking the case for a ban when the moratorium expires.

In the interim, I vote strongly in favor of the moratorium over the alternative proposal of regulation. First, because I am keenly aware of the power of the scientific imperative to breach frontiers of ethics, and deeply distrustful of the ability of society to resist those scientific imperatives. I am highly skeptical about the ultimate efficacy of regulation in preventing the breaching of further moral barriers.

And second, because regulation is really just a nicely confectured way of saying that we are prepared as a society today to utterly abolish a crucial moral barrier, namely, the prohibition of the creation of human embryos solely for the purpose of experimentation.

That is a serious moral barrier. The argument that we already crossed that barrier when we permitted the use of discarded embryos from IVF clinics for stem-cell research is simple sophistry.* Creating human embryos solely for their exploitation in research and therapy is new. It is dangerous. It is something that we will live to regret. A moratorium will prevent that for now, and allow a restatement of the case for its unwisdom and its danger when the issue is later reconsidered.

I support the moratorium on research cloning for several additional reasons. First, because the impasse on research cloning has led to congressional failure to enact any anti-cloning legislation. That is absurd. There is a unanimous national feeling that reproductive cloning should be banned. Our proposal provides a compromise that both sides can embrace so that cloning legislation can be passed.

------

* As I elaborate in my memo to Council Members, reprinted below.

.

Second, for those who support regulation, the moratorium is the only effective way to move toward serious regulation. The vague call for regulation, made by proponents of Position Two, has no political traction. None of the relevant players has any incentive to prepare the regulations. The scientific community is largely opposed to any interference in this research. And while people are dithering, the cloning research in the private biotech industries will put facts on the ground that will be difficult to challenge. Only a moratorium can test the good faith of those who say they want regulation. Moreover, Position Two does not explicitly say that the existence of the strict regulations it calls for is a precondition for allowing the research to go forward. There is no talk here, as there was in the public Council sessions, that this proposal amounts to a de facto moratorium.

Third, this proposal does not abandon the strong anti-cloning position. It stops cloning at the very beginning, namely at the point of creating a cloned embryo. It is thus much stronger than the pseudo-ban on cloning proposed by those who want regulation, which would block only implantation.

A ban on reproductive cloning and a moratorium on research cloning allows the country to clearly express itself: definitively make law regarding reproductive cloning and at least temporarily prevent the launching of an industry whose business is the manufacture of (cloned) human embryos purely for experimentation. And it allows the country to engage now in a serious and extended debate on the virtues and pitfalls of such an enterprise, on the promise and problems of regulation, and, ultimately, on the question of not only where these cells come from, but where these cells are taking us.

I include here a memo that I circulated to Council Members during our deliberations*:

*   *   *

The conquest of rejection is one of the principal rationales for research cloning. But there is reason to doubt this claim on scientific grounds. There is some empirical evidence in mice that cloned tissue may be rejected anyway (possibly because a clone contains a small amount of foreign—mitochondrial—DNA derived from the egg into which it was originally injected). Moreover, enormous advances are being made elsewhere in combating tissue rejection. The science of immune rejection is much more mature than the science of cloning. By the time we figure out how to do safe and reliable research cloning, the rejection problem

---

* A longer version of this argument appears in my article, "Crossing Lines," *The New Republic*, April 29, 2002, pp. 20-23.

may well be solved. And finally, there are less problematic alternatives—such as adult stem cells—that offer a promising alternative to cloning because they present no problem of tissue rejection and raise none of cloning's moral conundrums.

These scientific considerations raise serious questions about the efficacy of, and thus the need for, research cloning. But there is a stronger case to be made. Even if the scientific objections are swept aside, even if research cloning is as doable and promising as its advocates contend, there are other reasons to pause.

The most obvious is this: Research cloning is an open door to reproductive cloning. Banning the production of cloned babies while permitting the production of cloned embryos makes no sense. If you have factories all around the country producing embryos for research and commerce, it is inevitable that someone will implant one in a woman (or perhaps in some artificial medium in the farther future) and produce a human clone. What then? A law banning reproductive cloning but permitting research cloning would then make it a crime not to destroy that fetus—an obvious moral absurdity.

This is an irrefutable point and the reason alone to vote for the total ban on cloning. Philosophically, however, it is a showstopper. It lets us off too early and too easy. It keeps us from facing the deeper question: Is there anything about research cloning that in and of itself makes it morally problematic?

Objection I: Intrinsic Worth

For some people, life begins at conception. And not just life—if life is understood to mean a biologically functioning organism, even a single cell is obviously alive—but personhood. If the first zygotic cell is owed all the legal and moral respect due a person, then there is nothing to talk about. Ensoulment starts with Day One and Cell One, and the idea of taking that cell or its successor cells apart to serve someone else's needs is abhorrent.

This is an argument of great moral force but little intellectual interest. Not because it may not be right. But because it is unprovable. It rests on metaphysics. Either you believe it or you don't. The discussion ends there.

I happen not to share this view. I do not believe personhood begins at conception. I do not believe a single cell has the moral or legal standing of a child. This is not to say that I do not stand in awe of the developing embryo, a creation of majestic beauty and mystery. But I stand in equal awe of the Grand Canyon, the spider's web, and quantum mechanics. Awe commands wonder, humility, appreciation. It does not command inviolability. I am quite prepared to shatter an atom, take down a spider's web, or dam a canyon for electricity. (Though we'd have to be very short on electricity before I'd dam the Grand.)

I do not believe the embryo is entitled to inviolability. But is it entitled to nothing? There is a great distance between inviolability, on the one hand, and mere "thingness," on the other. Many advocates of research cloning see nothing but thingness. That view justifies the most ruthless exploitation of the embryo. That view is dangerous.

Why? Three possible reasons. First, the Brave New World Factor: Research cloning gives man too much power for evil. Second, the Slippery Slope: The habit of embryonic violation is in and of itself dangerous. Violate the blastocyst today and every day, and the practice will inure you to violating the fetus or even the infant tomorrow. Third, Manufacture: The very act of creating embryos for the sole purpose of exploiting and then destroying them will ultimately predispose us to a ruthless utilitarianism about human life itself.

Objection II: The Brave New World Factor

The physicists at Los Alamos did not hesitate to penetrate, manipulate, and split uranium atoms on the grounds that uranium atoms possess intrinsic worth that entitled them to inviolability. Yet after the war, many fought to curtail atomic power. They feared the consequences of delivering such unfathomable power—and potential evil—into the hands of fallible human beings. Analogously, one could believe that the cloned blastocyst has little more intrinsic worth than the uranium atom and still be deeply troubled by the manipulation of the blastocyst because of the fearsome power it confers upon humankind.

The issue is leverage. Our knowledge of how to manipulate human genetics (or atomic nuclei) is still primitive. We could never construct ex nihilo a human embryo. It is an unfolding organism of unimaginable complexity that took nature three billion years to produce. It might take us less time to build it from scratch, but not much less. By that time, we as a species might have acquired enough wisdom to use it wisely. Instead, the human race in its infancy has stumbled upon a genie infinitely too complicated to create or even fully understand, but understandable enough to command and perhaps even control. And given our demonstrated unwisdom with our other great discovery—atomic power: As we speak, the very worst of humanity is on the threshold of acquiring the most powerful weapons in history—this is a fear and a consideration to be taken very seriously.

For example. Female human eggs seriously limit the mass production of cloned embryos. Extracting eggs from women is difficult, expensive, and potentially dangerous. The search is on, therefore, for a good alternative. Scientists have begun injecting human nuclei into the egg cells of animals. In 1996 Massachusetts scientists injected a human nucleus with a cow egg. Chinese scientists have fused a human fibroblast with a rabbit egg and have grown the resulting embryo to the blastocyst stage. We have no idea what grotesque results might come from such interspecies clonal experiments.

In October 2000 the first primate containing genes from another species was born (a monkey with a jellyfish gene). In 1995 researchers in Texas produced headless mice. In 1997 researchers in Britain produced headless tadpoles. In theory, headlessness might be useful for organ transplantation. One can envision, in a world in which embryos are routinely manufactured, the production of headless clones—subhuman creatures with usable human organs but no head, no brain, no consciousness to identify them with the human family.

The heart of the problem is this: Nature, through endless evolution, has produced cells with totipotent power. We are about to harness that power for crude human purposes. That should give us pause. Just around the corner lies the logical by-product of such power: human-animal hybrids, partly developed human bodies for use as parts, and other horrors imagined—Huxley's Deltas and Epsilons—and as yet un imagined. This is the Brave New World Factor. Its grounds for objecting to this research are not about the beginnings of life, but about the ends; not the origin of these cells, but their destiny; not where we took these magnificent cells from, but where they are taking us.

Objection III: The Slippery Slope

The other prudential argument is that once you start tearing apart blastocysts, you get used to tearing apart blastocysts. And whereas now you'd only be doing that at the seven-day stage, when most people would look at this tiny clump of cells on the head of a pin and say it is not inviolable, it is inevitable that some scientist will soon say: Give me just a few more weeks to work with it and I could do wonders.

That will require quite a technological leap because the blastocyst will not develop as a human organism unless implanted in the uterus. That means that to go beyond that seven-day stage you'd have to implant this human embryo either in an animal uterus or in some fully artificial womb.

Both possibilities may be remote, but they are real. And then we'll have a scientist saying: Give me just a few more months with this embryo, and I'll have actual kidney cells, brain cells, pancreatic cells that I can transplant back into the donor of the clone and cure him. Scientists at Advanced Cell Technology in Massachusetts have already gone past that stage in animals. They have taken cloned cow embryos past the blastocyst stage, taken tissue from the more developed cow fetus, and reimplanted it back into the donor animal.

The scientists' plea to do the same in humans will be hard to ignore. Why grow the clone just to the blastocyst stage, destroy it, pull out the inner cell mass, grow stem cells out of that, propagate them in the laboratory, and then try chemically or otherwise to tweak them into becoming kidney cells or brain cells or islet cells? This is Rube Goldberg. Why not just allow that beautiful embryonic machine, created by nature and far more sophisticated than our crude techniques, to develop unmolested? Why not let the blastocyst grow into a fetus that possesses the kinds of differentiated tissue that we could then use for curing the donor?

Scientifically, this would make sense. Morally, we will have crossed the line between tearing apart a mere clump of cells and tearing apart a recognizable human fetus. And at that point, it would be an even smaller step to begin carving up seven- and eight-month-old fetuses with more perfectly formed organs to alleviate even more pain and suffering among the living. We will, slowly and by increments, have gone from stem cells to embryo farms to factories with fetuses in various stages of development and humanness, hanging (metaphorically) on meat hooks waiting to be cut open to be used by the already born.

We would all be revolted if a living infant or developed fetus were carved up for parts. Should we build a fence around that possibility by prohibiting any research on even the very earliest embryonic clump of cells? Is the only way to avoid the slide never to mount the slippery slope at all? On this question, I am personally agnostic. If I were utterly convinced that we would never cross the seven-day line, then I would have no objection on these grounds to such research on the inner cell mass of a blastocyst. The question is: Can we be sure? This is not a question of principle; it is a question of prudence. It is almost a question of psychological probability. No one yet knows the answer.

Objection IV: Manufacture

Note that while, up to now, I have been considering arguments against research cloning, they are all equally applicable to embryonic research done on a normal—i.e., noncloned—embryo. If the question is tearing up the blastocyst, there is no intrinsic moral difference between a two-parented embryo derived from a sperm and an egg and a single-parented embryo derived from a cloned cell. Thus the various arguments against this research—the intrinsic worth of the embryo, the prudential consideration that we might create monsters, or the prudential consideration that we might become monsters in exploiting post-embryonic forms of human life (fetuses or even children)—are identical to the arguments for and against stem-cell research.

These arguments are serious—serious enough to banish the insouciance of the scientists who consider anyone questioning their work to be a Luddite—yet, in my view, insufficient to justify a legal ban on stem-cell research (as with stem cells from discarded embryos in fertility clinics). I happen not to believe that either personhood or ensoulment occurs at conception. I think we need to be apprehensive about what evil might arise from the power of stem-cell research, but that apprehension alone, while justifying vigilance and regulation, does not justify a ban on the practice. And I believe that given the good that might flow from stem-cell research, we should first test the power of law and custom to enforce the seven-day blastocyst line for embryonic exploitation before assuming that such a line could never hold.

This is why I support stem-cell research (using leftover embryos from fertility clinics) and might support research cloning were it not for one other aspect that is unique to it. In research cloning, the embryo is created with the explicit intention of its eventual destruction. That is a given because not to destroy the embryo would be to produce a cloned child. If you are not permitted to grow the embryo into a child, you are obliged at some point to destroy it.

Deliberately creating embryos for eventual and certain destruction means the launching of an entire industry of embryo manufacture. It means the routinization, the commercialization, the commodification of the human embryo. The bill that would legalize research cloning essentially sanctions, licenses, and protects the establishment of a most ghoulish enterprise: the creation of nascent human life for the sole purpose of its exploitation and destruction.

How is this morally different from simply using discarded embryos from in vitro fertilization (IVF) clinics? Some have suggested that it is not, that to oppose research cloning is to oppose IVF and any stem-cell research that comes out of IVF. The claim is made that because in IVF there is a high probability of destruction of the embryo, it is morally equivalent to research cloning. But this is plainly not so. In research cloning there is not a high probability of destruction; there is 100 percent probability. Because every cloned embryo must be destroyed, it is nothing more than a means to someone else's end.

In IVF, the probability of destruction may be high, but it need not necessarily be. You could have a clinic that produces only a small number of embryos, and we know of many cases of multiple births resulting from multiple embryo implantation. In principle, one could have IVF using only a single embryo and thus involving no deliberate embryo destruction at all. In principle, that is impossible in research cloning.

Furthermore, a cloned embryo is created to be destroyed and used by others. An IVF embryo is created to develop into a child. One cannot disregard intent in determining morality. Embryos are created in IVF to serve reproduction. Embryos are created in research cloning to serve, well, research. If certain IVF embryos were designated as "helper embryos" that would simply aid an anointed embryo in turning into a child, then we would have an analogy to cloning. But, in fact, we don't know which embryo is anointed in IVF. They are all created to have a chance of survival. And they are all equally considered an end.

Critics counter that this ends-and-means argument is really obfuscation, that both procedures make an instrument of the embryo. In cloning, the creation and destruction of the embryo is a means to understanding or curing disease. In IVF, the creation of the embryo is a means of satisfying a couple's need for a child. They are both just means to ends.

But it makes no sense to call an embryo a means to the creation of a child. The creation of a child is the destiny of an embryo. To speak of an embryo as a means to creating a child empties the word "means" of content. The embryo in IVF is a stage in the development of a child; it is no more a means than a teenager is a means to the adult he or she later becomes. In contrast, an embryo in research cloning is pure means. Laboratory pure.

And that is where we must draw the line. During the great debate on stem-cell research, a rather broad consensus was reached (among those not committed to "intrinsic worth" rendering all embryos inviolable) that stem-cell research could be morally justified because the embryos destroyed for their possibly curative stem cells were derived from fertility clinics and thus were going to be discarded anyway. It was understood that human embryos should not be created solely for the purpose of being dismembered and then destroyed for the benefit of others. Indeed, when Senator Bill Frist made his impassioned presentation on the floor of the Senate supporting stem-cell research, he included among his conditions a total ban on creating human embryos just to be stem-cell farms.

Where cloning for research takes us decisively beyond stem-cell research is in sanctioning the manufacture of the human embryo. You can try to regulate embryonic research to prohibit the creation of Brave New World monsters; you can build fences on the slippery slope, regulating how many days you may grow an embryo for research; but once you countenance the very creation of human embryos for no other purpose than for their parts, you have crossed a moral frontier.

Research cloning is the ultimate in conferring thingness up on the human embryo. It is the ultimate in desensitization. And as such, it threatens whatever other fences and safeguards we might erect around embryonic research. The problem, one could almost say, is not what cloning does to the embryo, but what it does to us. Except that, once cloning has changed us, it will inevitably enable further assaults on human dignity. Creating a human embryo just so it can be used and then destroyed undermines the very foundation of the moral prudence that informs the entire enterprise of genetic research: the idea that, while a human embryo may not be a person, it is not nothing. Because if it is nothing, then everything is permitted. And if everything is permitted, then there are no fences, no safeguards, no bottom.

CHARLES KRAUTHAMMER

*   *   *

Statement of Dr. McHugh

I am concerned that section (g) of Part I of Chapter Eight does not adequately describe my views about somatic cell nuclear transfer (SCNT), expressed at several meetings of the Council. That section says, "[P]roposals to engage in cloning-for-biomedical-research necessarily endorse the creation of human (cloned) embryos *solely for the purpose of such research*. Public policy that specifically promoted this research would thus *explicitly and officially approve* crossing a moral boundary." (Italics in the text.) I believe (1) those words imply that the prime effect of SCNT is the creation of a new individual human being and (2) that implication prejudges the problem before us and does not comport to my opinion of this matter.

I hold that SCNT rests on a major discovery in cellular biology, the implications of which need much more discussion and debate than it receives in Chapter Eight (and especially in section (g)). With this discovery we now know that every one of our somatic cells not only has a full complement of our genes but as well that every one of our somatic cells, if manipulated in a particular fashion, has the power to recapitulate in growth its own beginnings.

When a technician takes a donor's somatic cell and proceeds with it to follow the method of somatic cell nuclear transplantation, he or she evokes an intrinsic program present within that nucleus that brings about cellular multiplication and differentiation. One need not hold that a new and unique human individual starts up immediately as these cells are made and multiply. One could see this process as an engineered culturing of cells from the somatic nucleus that recapitulates embryonic development but rests upon a potential for growth and replication resident in and intrinsic to all somatic cells. The cellular products are direct extensions of the donor as with other forms of tissue culture and as such have some licit potentials for further use.

I agree with those who say that my argument—that the products of SCNT and the products of impregnation are crucially different—places a strong emphasis on origins of these products and less emphasis on potentials that we deplore. But I would hold that the section (g) from Part I of Chapter Eight places all the emphasis on potential and no emphasis on origins. It thus ignores the fact that an overemphasis on potential would lead us to the unreasonable position that since every one of our somatic cells has "potential" for producing a human, it should receive some reverence. I believe that in our presentation to the American people we must acknowledge that some of the arguments in favor of the use of SCNT rest upon the view that what is emerging here are cells and not human beings. This very fundamental disagreement should be thoroughly aired, as it carries with it quite different policy implications.

PAUL MCHUGH

Statement of Dr. May

Substantial moral debate on cloning-for-biomedical-research focuses on the question as to whether the preimplanted embryo is "one of us" or not. The group in favor of unregulated research would define "one of us" narrowly in order to exclude the microscopic material in the petri dish from "one of us." Therefore we can do with it what we will. Proponents of a ban define "one of us" broadly to include the preimplanted embryo. Therefore they would refuse to clone/kill a preimplanted embryo used in research, even at the expense of the relief that successful research might offer some patients who are seriously impaired or face premature death. Both parties seek to escape the stigma (and perhaps the regulatory burdens) that might accompany therapy that owed something to "one of us."

However, there is a way of thinking about the preimplanted embryo that does not rely on the inclusionary/exclusionary language of "one of us." The somewhat awkward language of the intermediate status of the embryo (neither a mere thing nor a full human being) both *permits* research but also *requires* regulation. The status of the preimplanted embryo permits research because it does not hold such a claim on us as to ban a line of inquiry that might thwart grave human suffering and premature death. However, the *source* of this research in the human argues for the necessity of regulations. The preimplanted embryo is more than a yard lot of building materials; it is a cluster of cells moving toward, if implanted, nourished, and protected, a human life. In removing it, through research, from the circle of life, we cannot remove it from the circle of human indebtedness.

This position has powerful implications for the *content* as well as the necessity of regulations. Most discussion has centered on regulations as they might bear on the generation of knowledge and therapies (for example, the protection of women as the source of eggs, the time limit on research to a fourteen-day period before the onset of the neural streak, the development of licensing and monitoring procedures, and extending the scope of regulations to private as well as publicly funded projects). However, the acceptance of a human source for the conduct of this research has equally powerful consequences for the distribution of knowledge and therapies. Gratefully accepting a human source that makes possible the conduct of this research requires the most inclusive destination of its fruits in the common good. The element of gift in origin requires common human access to benefits. It does not permit the capture of knowledge and benefits in such a way as to thwart their eventual arrival to all in need.

WILLIAM F. MAY

* * *

Statement of Professor Meilaender

Like some of my colleagues on the Council, I believe that a ban on all forms of human cloning (including a ban on what in this report is called cloning-for-biomedical-research) would be the optimal policy for this Council to recommend and for our society to adopt. Nevertheless, because other Council Members who have serious moral reservations about human cloning are not at this time prepared to recommend a permanent ban on all human cloning, we have joined with them to support a policy that would ban cloning-to-produce-children and would place a four-year moratorium on cloning-for-biomedical-research. Even if the policy I regard as optimal is for now impossible, we need not settle for no policy at all. Nor should we think of the majority recommendation as simply a compromise position. On the contrary, we have found genuine—though only partial—agreement with some of our colleagues on the Council, and I prefer to try to use and build on that partial agreement than to act as if it were unimportant or insignificant. Were the majority recommendation enacted into law, it would prohibit all human cloning (whether publicly or privately funded) for four years. That would be a considerable achievement. It would give us a period in which the optimal policy was in place, during which time we would hope that further moral debate and advances in alternative forms of research (that would not involve human cloning or destruction of embryos) would persuade others to continue that optimal policy indefinitely.

In the Council's deliberations, those who oppose all human cloning have worked very hard to respect and acknowledge the views of Council Members with whom we disagree or do not fully agree. In particular, the following points are worth noting:

(a) For the sake of continued conversation, we have acquiesced in terminology that some of us do not fully accept and that to some extent distorts our position. That is, any human cloning is morally objectionable, and there is for some of us no crucial moral divide between cloning-for-biomedical-research and cloning-to-produce-children. Put differently, research cloning is also reproductive cloning, since it brings into existence a new human being (in the very earliest stages of developing human life). Agreeing to converse in terms that do not fully acknowledge this has inevitably been problematic; nevertheless, we have accepted this burden so that the Council's work could proceed. I believe that the definitions of cloning-for-biomedical-research and cloning-to-produce-children given at the end of Chapter Three of the Council's report make clear that, however the proximate or ultimate purposes of those engaged in cloning may differ, the nature of the act remains the same.

(b) In supporting a proposed four-year moratorium on cloning-for-biomedical-research (even though some of us are quite prepared to support a permanent ban) we have sought to make common cause with those Council Members who worry more about cloning-to-produce-children than about cloning-for-biomedical-research and for whom control of the latter is chiefly a means to control of the former. I myself incline to think, on the contrary, that an industry of routinized embryo cloning (which would be the inevitable result of approval of cloning-for-biomedical-research) would be an even greater moral evil than the gestation and birth of a cloned human being. Nevertheless, recognizing that some colleagues on the Council who support a moratorium do not yet share this view, others of us have chosen to endorse the partial agreement that we do now share.

(c) We have accepted in good faith the assertion—and it has seldom been more than an assertion—that advocates of cloning-for-biomedical-research have a principled commitment to drawing a line at a very early point in embryonic development and permitting no research beyond that point. We have accepted this in good faith even though we have been offered no coherent argument to support the "developmental" view of human status put forward by cloning proponents. Other Members of the Council have offered a variety of arguments against that view. We have offered evidence that embryologists do not make the sort of distinction on which cloning proponents rely. We have noted that the embryo's "potential" is something actual, something present in the developing human being, and that it is a misuse of the idea of potential to describe the embryo as merely a potential human being. We have argued that, while it is true that we would be unlikely to feel the same grief at the death of an embryo as we do at the death of a child, this hardly means that the embryo's life should not be protected. We have noted that criteria for "protectability" offered by at least one Council member (namely, the presence of brain activity) would clearly permit research to a point well beyond the development of the early embryo. Indeed, I do not think that the Council has been fully willing to take up the question of the moral status of the embryo. Nevertheless, despite the belief of some of us that the morality of human cloning probably cannot be addressed satisfactorily without doing so, we have agreed that the Council must examine the morality of cloning in ways alert to the many other important moral issues it also raises.

(d) Most of all, we have been willing to join in this report's majority recommendation of a policy that would prohibit cloning-to-produce-children and prohibit for four years all cloning-for-biomedical-research, even though such a policy is not, in our view, the optimal one. We have concurred in this recommendation in order to join with some Council Members who, because of their moral concerns about human cloning, endorse a moratorium for reasons somewhat different from ours. I, for instance, specifically decline to think of a moratorium as simply providing time to put in place regulations—after which cloning-for-biomedical-research could proceed. For me a moratorium is good because it prohibits all human cloning for four years and provides opportunity to continue the argument and the research that may, one hopes, make the case against cloning still more persuasive four years hence. Although some of us would favor a ban on all cloning, including cloning-for-biomedical-research, we have recognized that such a policy proposal would, in effect, have said to fellow Council Members who, for their own different reasons, support a moratorium: "We're not prepared to continue this discussion." Rather than adopt such a position, we have been willing to support a position we regard as good even if less than optimal. As I noted above, however, this is not simply a compromise position. On the contrary, it is a partial agreement which may, I hope, give rise to still greater agreement in the future.

Finally, I note the following about the moral (and not simply the policy) aspects of the human cloning debate:

(a) A number of Council Members, of whom I am one, hold that the human embryo is fully deserving of our moral respect and that such respect is incompatible with its deliberate destruction in research. That judgment about the status of the human embryo (whether cloned or resulting from union of egg and sperm) is not, so far as I can see, based on our religious beliefs. We have taken seriously what the science of embryology teaches us. We have taken seriously what careful philosophical reasoning about the meaning of "potentiality" teaches us. We have taken seriously the lessons of human history in which the limits of our sympathy for fellow human beings who seem "different" from us have more than once had to be overcome in order to learn a more inclusive and egalitarian respect for human life. This does not mean, for me at least, that religious belief should play no role here. On the contrary, Jews worship a Lord who favors the widow and the orphan, who teaches us to speak on behalf of those no one else defends. And Christians worship a crucified God who has himself accepted vulnerability. Instructed by our religious traditions, we may see in the weakest and most vulnerable of human beings—those unable to speak in their own behalf—special objects of our care. Such care for the vulnerable seems to me incompatible with an industry of routine manufacture, use, and destruction of cloned embryos—even if the goal is to help others who are also vulnerable.

(b) The position of those who support cloning-for-biomedical-research (while opposing cloning-to-produce-children) amounts, in effect, to criminalizing the implantation of cloned embryos. Nothing could be more revealing of the moral underpinnings of their position. In their view, moral status is conferred not by belonging to the human species but by the will and choice of some human beings (those like us who are stronger and in control). We cannot pretend that being *un*implanted is somehow a natural fact about an embryo; on the contrary, it is what we choose. First we produce the cloned human embryo, then we decide to use it for our purposes in research rather than to implant it, and then we argue that until implanted it lacks the capacity for continued development. This reasoning is specious, it should be rejected, and it can find no support in the definitions given at the close of Chapter Three of this report.

(c) Because the defense of cloning-for-biomedical-research rests ultimately upon a view that the will and choice of some confers moral status on others, and because no coherent defense of the "developmental" approach to human dignity and worth has been offered by proponents of research cloning, I think it very unlikely that research—if allowed to proceed—can really be confined to the early blastocyst. With no principled reasons to place limits on our will, and with the likelihood that more developed embryos or fetuses will actually be much more useful for researchers, I doubt whether the momentum of cloning research can be stopped in any way other than by stopping all human cloning. Indeed, I suspect that, if cloning-for-biomedical-research proceeds, the distinction between cloning-for-biomedical-research and cloning-to-produce-children will come to seem artificial. Having accustomed ourselves to use cloning techniques to shape and mold the next generation, we will be hard-pressed to explain why we should not, in fact, exercise an even fuller control by cloning-to-produce-children. Our earlier opposition to it will seem to have been merely sentimental.

I am happy, therefore, to join with other colleagues on the Council in recommending a policy that would prohibit for at least four years all human cloning, whether for the purpose only of research or for the additional purpose of producing children, but it is imperative to emphasize that this good policy is less than optimal. We should hope that four years from now our society will be able to do still better.

GILBERT C. MEILAENDER

* * *

Statement of Dr. Rowley

Support for Proposal Two

During the deliberations of the President's Council on Bioethics, we asked many questions about the comparative usefulness of embryonic compared with adult human stem cells to treat a host of fatal and non-fatal but debilitating diseases. We never received a clear answer; thus the role of stem cell treatment is largely based on promise, rather than on persuasive evidence of efficacy. Given the intense interest of scientists in this research problem for at least a decade, the public can reasonably ask why we do not have convincing data on the use of embryonic stem cells to treat diabetes, Parkinson's disease and other medical problems?

The answer is shockingly clear! American scientists have been prevented from working on these very critical problems because of a ban on any federally funded research using cells from human embryos. Progress in our understanding of human diseases and the development of effective treatment for these diseases has come largely from federally funded research, primarily supported through NIH. Thus, a consequence of the present Congressional ban (instituted in 1994 after an NIH panel established guidelines and oversight to allow such research) has been that the only research on the development of embryonic stem cell lines and on the use of embryonic cells has been limited to private and for-profit ventures. Not only are these efforts relatively small as compared with those funded by NIH, the results are largely hidden from the general scientific community and the benefits are likely to be available to the public on a very restricted basis, usually based on the ability to pay whatever price is asked. The effect of extending and expanding this moratorium will be to maintain our ignorance by preventing any research for four more years; this proposal will force American scientists who have private funding to stop their research. It will also accelerate the scientific "brain-drain" to more enlightened countries.

The recent publication of reports on the plasticity of human stem cells from adult bone marrow has raised the possibility that the problem is solved, that we do not need stem cells derived from embryos. However, even Dr. Catherine Verfaillie (author of one such report) emphasizes the need for research on embryonic stem cells to complement work on adult stem cells. Will adult stem cells have the same unlimited capacity for renewal as is present in embryonic cells? Will embryonic and adult stem cells both be suitable for somatic cell nuclear transfer? Will embryonic or adult stem cells be more amenable to manipulation to reduce the problem of immune rejection? These are just a few of the critical questions that are urgently in need of answers – answers that NIH is prohibited from allowing American scientists to answer.

As summarized here, it is clear that there is an urgent need immediately to fund research on the actual potential of human embryonic stem cells to treat human disease. However, it is equally clear that research using cells from human embryos requires great sensitivity and careful thought. It is thus appropriate to accompany the lifting of the NIH ban with the simultaneous implementation of an appropriate regulatory mechanism. It is important to emphasize that every US academic institution has an Institutional Review Board in place, whose function is to review all research related to human subjects before a grant can be submitted to any agency for funding; this ensures that the research proposal protects the health, safety and privacy of the individuals involved in the project. In 1998, the NIH Director established a task force to review the policy regarding stem cell research. This task force developed Guidelines for Pluripotent Stem Cell Research which were approved after extensive public comment (more than 50,000 responses) and which were published in the Federal Registry, August 2000. The task force proposed the establishment of The Human Embryonic Research Board. This Board would represent a broad constituency including consumers, ethicists, lawyers, as well as scientists knowledgeable in all aspects of human and animal embryonic stem cell research appointed by the Secretary of HHS. Thus there is no need to delay research until a Board is in place because the design of the Board is already in place.

Our ignorance is profound; the potential for important medical advances is very great. We must remove the current impediments to this critical research. Congress should lift the ban and establish a broadly constituted regulatory board, NOW.

JANET D. ROWLEY

*   *   *

Statement of Professor Sandel

After six months of searching ethical and scientific inquiry, a majority of this Council has rejected a ban on cloning-for-biomedical-research of the kind passed by the House of Representatives last year. Among those of us who reject a ban, some prefer a moratorium, while others would permit such research to proceed subject to regulation. (See table in Chapter Eight.)

I will first give my reasons for concluding that cloning-for-biomedical-research should not be banned, and then explain why I believe such research should be permitted subject to regulation.

Any ethical analysis of cloning-for-biomedical-research must address the moral status of the human embryo. Before turning to that question, however, it is important to place cloning-for-biomedical-research in the broader context of embryonic stem cell research. Some who find cloning-for-biomedical-research morally objectionable support stem cell research that uses spare embryos left over from fertility clinics. They argue that it is wrong to create embryos for research (whether cloned or non-cloned) but morally acceptable to use excess embryos created for reproduction, since these "spare" embryos would otherwise be discarded. But this distinction is not persuasive. If it is wrong to carry out stem cell research on embryos created for research, it is wrong to carry out any embryonic stem cell research.

Those who oppose the creation of embryos for stem cell research but support research on embryos left over from in vitro fertilization (IVF) clinics beg the question whether those IVF "spares" should have been created in the first place: if it is immoral to create and sacrifice embryos for the sake of curing or treating devastating diseases, why isn't it also objectionable to create and discard spare IVF embryos for the sake of treating infertility? After all, both practices serve worthy ends, and curing diseases such as Parkinson's, Alzheimer's, and diabetes is at least as important as enabling infertile couples to have genetically related children.

Those who would distinguish the sacrifice of embryos in IVF from the sacrifice of embryos in stem cell research might reply as follows: the fertility doctor who creates excess embryos does not know which embryos will ultimately be sacrificed, and does not intend the death of any; but the scientist who deliberately creates an embryo for stem cell research knows the embryo will die, for to carry out the research is necessarily to destroy the embryo.

But it is hard to see the moral difference between a practice that typically sacrifices embryos (by the tens of thousands, in the case of the IVF industry) and one that inevitably does so. If IVF as currently practiced in the United States is morally permissible, its justification does not rest on the idea that the sacrifice it entails is only typical, not inevitable. It rests instead on the idea that the good achieved outweighs the loss, and that the loss is not of a kind that violates the respect embryos are due. This is the same moral test that must be met to justify the creation of embryos for stem cell research and regenerative medicine.

Comparing the range of practices that sacrifice embryos clarifies the stakes: if cloning-for-biomedical-research is morally wrong, then so is all embryonic stem cell research, and so is any version of IVF that creates and discards excess embryos. If, morally speaking, these practices stand or fall together, it remains to ask whether they stand or fall. The answer to that question depends on the moral status of the embryo.

There are three possible ways of conceiving the moral status of the embryo—as a thing, as a person, or as something in between. To regard an embryo as a mere thing, open to any use we may desire or devise, misses its significance as nascent human life. One need not regard an embryo as a full human person in order to believe that it is due a certain respect. Personhood is not the only warrant for respect; we consider it a failure of respect when a thoughtless hiker carves his initials in an ancient sequoia—not because we regard the sequoia as a person, but because we consider it a natural wonder worthy of appreciation and awe—modes of regard inconsistent with treating it as a billboard or defacing it for the sake of petty vanity. To respect the old growth forest does not mean that no tree may ever be felled or harvested for human purposes. Respecting the forest may be consistent with using it. But the purposes should be weighty and appropriate to the wondrous nature of the thing.

One way to oppose a degrading, objectifying stance toward nascent human life is to attribute full personhood to the embryo. Because this view is associated with the religious doctrine that personhood begins at conception, it is sometimes said to be a matter of faith that lies beyond rational argument. But it is a mistake to assume that religiously informed beliefs are mere dogmas, beyond the reach of critical reflection. One way of respecting a religious conviction is to take it seriously—to probe and explore its moral implications.

The notion that the embryo is a person carries far-reaching consequences, some of which emerged in the course of this Council's deliberations. One is that harvesting stem cells from a seven-day-old blastocyst is as morally abhorrent as harvesting organs from a baby. This is a bold and principled claim, even if deeply at odds with most people's moral intuitions. But the implications do not stop there. If the equal moral status view is correct, then the penalty provided in recent anti-cloning legislation—a million dollar fine and ten years in prison—is woefully inadequate. If embryonic stem cell research is morally equivalent to yanking organs from babies, it should be treated as a grisly form of murder, and the scientist who performs it should face life imprisonment or the death penalty.

A further source of difficulty for the equal moral status view lies in the fact that, in natural pregnancies, at least half of all embryos either fail to implant or are otherwise lost. If natural procreation entails the loss of some number of embryos for every successful birth, then perhaps we should worry less about the loss of embryos that occurs in IVF and in stem cell research. It might be replied that a high rate of infant mortality does not justify infanticide. But the way we respond to the natural loss of embryos suggests that we do not regard these events as the moral or religious equivalent of infant mortality. Otherwise, wouldn't we carry out the same burial rituals and the same rites of mourning for the loss of an embryo that we observe for the death of a child?

The conviction that the embryo is a person derives support not only from certain religious doctrines but also from the Kantian assumption that the moral universe is divided in binary terms: everything is either a person, worthy of respect, or a thing, open to use. But as the sequoia example suggests, this dualism is overdrawn.

The way to combat the instrumentalizing impulse of modern technology and commerce is not to insist on an all-or-nothing ethic of respect for persons that consigns the rest of life to a utilitarian calculus. Such an ethic risks turning every moral question into a battle over the bounds of personhood. We would do better to cultivate a more expansive appreciation of life as a gift that commands our reverence and restricts our use. Human cloning to create designer babies is the ultimate expression of the hubris that marks the loss of reverence for life as a gift. But stem cell research to cure debilitating diseases, using seven-day-old blastocysts, cloned or uncloned, is a noble exercise of our human ingenuity to promote healing and to play our part in repairing the given world.

Those who warn of slippery slopes, embryo farms, and the commodification of ova and zygotes are right to worry but wrong to assume that cloning-for-biomedical-research necessarily opens us to these dangers. Rather than ban stem cell cloning and other forms of embryo research, we should allow them to proceed subject to regulations that embody the moral restraint appropriate to the mystery of the first stirrings of human life. Such regulations should include licensing requirements for embryo research projects and fertility clinics, restrictions on the commodification of eggs and sperm, and measures to prevent proprietary interests from monopolizing access to stem cell lines. This approach, it seems to me, offers the best hope of avoiding the wanton use of nascent human life and making these biomedical advances a blessing for health rather than an episode in the erosion of our human sensibilities.

MICHAEL J. SANDEL

*   *   *

Statement of Professor Wilson

Regulated Cloning-for-Biomedical-Research

I would allow regulated biomedical research on cloned embryos provided the blastocyst is no more than fourteen days old and would not allow implantation in a uterus, human or animal.

I take this position because I believe that research on human blastocysts may have substantial medical value in finding ways of improving human life. As our report indicates, such research may help doctors deal with Parkinson's disease, Alzheimer's disease, juvenile diabetes, and spinal cord injury. Members of the Council disagree as to how best to do that research.

The group that favors a moratorium on the use of cloned embryos for such research may think that the study of adult stem cells or in vitro fertilized eggs that are not used to impregnate a woman will produce all the knowledge we need to discover whether stem cells have therapeutic value. The other group, of which I am a part, favors regulated research on cloned embryos because it believes that all sources of stem cells, including those produced from cloned blastocysts, must be studied if we are to discover whether great medical advances are possible. That is because the use of cloned blastocysts may be the only important way of overcoming the problems of immune rejection and learning more about genetic diseases. If substantial medical benefit can be had from research, then it is unlikely that those benefits will derive from studying only stem cells derived from adult tissue or from leftover IVF eggs. To follow the policy recommended by the majority of this Council would be to do research with one hand tied behind our backs.

Moreover, I do not think there is any moral difference between a fertilized egg created in an in vitro fertilization clinic and one created by cloning an embryo. Both eggs are deliberately produced by scientific intervention and both (except for the IVF egg used to impregnate a woman) are destroyed.

Having said that there is no moral difference between these two sources of eggs does not mean, I believe, that using either kind of egg does not raise important and difficult moral questions. Every human begins as a fertilized egg, even though not every fertilized egg becomes a human. But the issue before us is not whether any human life should be destroyed but whether every fertilized egg should be preserved. To oppose the willful destruction of any fertilized egg is to oppose in vitro fertilization (since all fertilized eggs beyond that needed for successful implantation will be destroyed). Yet, in vitro procedures have produced (as of 1999) about thirty thousand babies for otherwise infertile couples. Initially, in vitro fertilizations were opposed by many who have since changed their minds, because the great benefits (many healthy new infants) so greatly outweighed the trivial costs (some tiny cells frozen or destroyed).

A fertilized cell has some moral worth, but much less than that of an implanted cell, and that has less than that of a fetus, and that less than that of a viable fetus, and that the same as of a newborn infant. My view is that people endow a thing with humanity when it appears, or even begins to appear, human; that is, when it resembles a human creature. The more an embryo resembles a person, the more claims it exerts on our moral feelings. Now this last argument has no religious or metaphysical meaning, but it accords closely, in my view, with how people view one another. It helps us understand why aborting a fetus in the twentieth week is more frightening than doing so in the first, and why so-called partial birth abortions are so widely opposed. And this view helps us understand why an elderly, comatose person lacking the ability to speak or act has more support from people than a seven-week-old fetus that also lacks the ability to speak or act.

Human worth grows as humanity becomes more apparent. In general, we are profoundly grieved by the death of a newborn, deeply distressed by the loss of a nearly born infant or a late-month miscarriage, and (for most but not all people) worried but not grieved by the abortion of a seven-week-old fetus. Our humanity, and thus the moral worth we assign to people, never leaves us even if many elements of it are later stripped away by age or disease.

This fact becomes evident when we ask a simple question: Do we assign the same moral blame to harvesting organs from a newborn infant and from a seven-day-old blastocyst? The great majority of people would be more outraged by doing the former than by doing the latter. A seven-day-old blastocyst that is no more than one millimeter in diameter and contains only a hundred or so largely undifferentiated cells does not make the same moral claims on us as does a live infant. Unless everyone who makes this distinction is wrong, then the moral status of a blastocyst is vastly less compelling than that of a neonate.

Some people believe that human life begins at conception and ought to be free from any human attack from that moment on. The difficulty with this rejoinder is that a large fraction (perhaps one-third or one-half) of fertilized cells fail to implant in the uterus or, if implanted, fail to develop into an embryo. Knowing this, one who offers this rejoinder would have to say that there is at best only a reasonable chance that the event of conception begins a human life.

But even blastocysts and leftover IVF eggs deserve some protection, because if society authorizes their destruction it has taken a dramatic and morally significant step. It has intervened in a profoundly important human process in ways that may lead future generations to take what may then appear to be the easy next steps, such as implanting a cloned embryo in a uterus or killing a fetus to extract some supposedly beneficial substance.

To avoid this, I favor federal regulations that would ban implanting a cloned embryo in any uterus, animal as well as human, and would insist that every cloned embryo raised in a glass dish exist for no more than fourteen days.

There is always some risk that allowing even strongly regulated research will create conditions that lead some scientists to ask for access to fertilized eggs beyond the blastocyst stage. But I do not believe we can object to this by making a generalized slippery slope argument, since virtually every medical procedure that involves entering or affecting the human body would also be liable to such an argument, a conclusion that would leave us (for example) without surgery. The slippery slope argument, stated baldly, would lead us to oppose allowing doctors to remove an inflamed appendix because they might later decide to remove a kidney, and after that a heart, and to oppose as well doctors prescribing a drug that will harm 0.5 percent of its recipients because we suspect that, once they do this, they will later insist on prescribing drugs that harm 1 percent, and then 10 percent, and possibly 50 percent of their patients. There may be good slippery slope arguments, but they cannot rest simply on the phrase "slippery slope"; they must also point clearly to a serious moral hazard and contain some reason for thinking that this hazard will become much more likely if we take the first step.

JAMES Q. WILSON

Made in the USA
Middletown, DE
19 December 2016